Atlas of Wound Healing

A Tissue Regeneration Approach

Editorial Board

Atlas of Wound Healing

A Tissue Regeneration Approach

SOHEILA S. KORDESTANI
Biomedical Engineering Faculty
Amirkabir University of Technology
Tehran, Iran

Managing Director
ChitoTech Inc., Tehran, Iran

ELSEVIER

Publisher: Dolores Meloni
Acquisition Editor: Charlotta Kryhl
Editorial Project Manager: Rebeka Henry
Production Project Manager: Kiruthika Govindaraju
Cover Designer: Miles Hitchen

3251 Riverport Lane
St. Louis, Missouri 63043

Working together
to grow libraries in
developing countries

www.elsevier.com • www.bookaid.org

Preface

The increasing incidence of wounds in the aging population, the rising prevalence of diabetes and thus diabetic foot ulcer, and the large number of other chronic wounds associated with diseases and abnormalities make it imperative to have a deeper understanding of wounds and develop a preventive approach in the first instance.

The new thinking in healthcare and the advent of advanced wound care modalities, which has become one of the major areas in regenerative medicine, has provided relatively better moist tissue environment, accelerated the inflammatory response, quality granulation tissue formation, and infection control during wound healing. Modern dressings provide an appropriate space to facilitate the cellular activities (i.e., migration and proliferation) and evoke the soluble mediators to regenerate the damaged tissues faster.

This Atlas of Wound is the outcome of approximately 14 years of dedicated efforts to collect the result of using advanced wound care modalities on a large number of patients of diverse ethnicities with different types of acute and chronic wounds of different etiologies. I hope it can be of benefit for medical community.

Acknowledgments

Preparing this "Atlas of Wound" was harder than I imagined. None of this would have been possible without ChitoTech nurses and wound care specialists working day and night on the wounds of many patients. Special thanks to Dr. Sami Abyaneh and Dr. Fayyazbakhsh, for taking this difficult task as editors, and our dedicated R&D team. I am also eternally grateful to the doctors, surgeons, and nurses in many hospitals throughout Iran for cooperating with us to use ChitoTech advanced wound dressings on the patients.

I would like to express my sincere gratitude to the following hospitals for their support:

- Imam Khomeini Hospital, Tehran, Iran
- Chamran Hospital, Tehran, Iran
- Shahid Motahari Burns Hospital, Tehran, Iran
- Shariati Hospital, Tehran, Iran
- Vali Asr subspecialty Hospital, Tehran, Iran
- Shohadaye Tajrish Hospital, Tehran, Iran
- Imam Reza Hospital—501 AJA, Tehran, Iran
- Masih Daneshvari Hospital, Tehran, Iran
- Rasoul Akram Hospital, Tehran, Iran
- Dr. Mo'eiri Hospital, Tehran, Iran
- Imam Reza hospital, Qom, Iran
- Gharazi Hospital, Sirjan, Kerman, Iran
- Imam Khomeini Hospital, Urmia, Iran
- Pasteur no Hospital, Tehran, Iran
- Naft Company Hospital, Tehran, Iran
- Sina Hospital, Tehran, Iran
- Loghman Hakim Hospital, Tehran, Iran
- Children's Medical Center, Tehran, Iran
- Shohadaye Haftome Tir Hospital, Tehran, Iran
- Firoozgar Hospital, Tehran, Iran
- State Welfare Organization of Iran (Jalaei Pour Clinic), Tehran, Iran
- Baharloo Hospital, Tehran, Iran
- Kashani Hospital, Tehran, Iran
- Bahrami Children Hospital, Tehran, Iran
- Razi Hospital, Tehran, Iran

Last but not least, I would like to thank my husband, my companion for that last 35 years, who have always supported me in every work I have done and my son and daughter for supporting me.

About the Author

Dr. Kordestani is a protein chemist, graduated from Leeds University in 1990, and worked as a research fellow at the Department of Medicine at Birmingham University. She has been working in the field of Wound Healing in Iran for the last 20 years. She is a faculty member and a lecturer in Biomedical Engineering Department at the Amirkabir University of Technology, and her primary teaching focus is on the topic of wound healing and the role of biomaterials, aimed at graduate students. She has extensive industry contacts as the founder of a knowledge-based company, manufacturing advanced wound care products. The biomaterial used in these products has been protected by five international and European patents.

List of Figures

List of Tables

Contents

Contents

CHAPTER 1

Introduction

The increasing incidence of wounds in the aging population, the rising prevalence of diabetes and thus diabetic leg ulcer, and the large number of other chronic wounds associated with diseases and abnormalities make it imperative to have a deeper understanding of wound and develop a preventive approach in the first instance.

When there is a wound, the surrounding tissues are damaged in the organ involved and the local environment within that organ is damaged; therefore, wound healing is a complex process involving many cell populations, the extracellular matrix, and soluble mediators such as growth factors and cytokines. To reduce the burden of wound in healthcare, it is necessary to have a deep understanding of pathophysiological processes of healing. Even more so it is essential to view wound healing as tissue healing and understand the interrelated processes taking place between cell–cell, cell–ECM (Extra Cellular Matrix), vascular tissues, and many biomolecules activated during the healing process.

Currently, several clinically proven strategies have been developed for wound treatment. Despite their relative effectiveness in wound healing, these strategies face multiple challenges including inadequate tissue repair, scar tissue formation without any skin appendages, limited vascularization, poor infection control, and high cost.

Tissue regeneration, as one of the major areas of regenerative medicine, has been developed to make up for donor tissue shortages, tissue replacement rejections, and delayed inflammation responses. Tissue regeneration strategies for wound healing have been focused on providing moisturized environments, accelerating the inflammatory response, quality granulation tissue formation, and infection control during tissue regeneration. Modern dressings provide an appropriate space to facilitate the cellular activities (i.e., migration and proliferation) and evoke the soluble mediators to regenerate the damaged tissues faster [1–4].

As everything in the world, including medical care systems, is becoming digitized, in this atlas a new technique for wound area measurement has been introduced: "HealApp" is a powerful cognitive mobile application, which measures the wound area quantitatively using artificial intelligence.

This atlas is the outcome of approximately 14 years of dedicated efforts on a large number of patients of diverse ethnicities with different types of wound and different etiologies. These wounds were healed using a brand of novel wound care products called "ChitoTech". These products are based on a natural biopolymer, chitosan.

PREVALENCE AND BURDEN OF WOUNDS

Owing to a significant increase in the global average life expectancy and hence, the age-related diseases and altered life style, the prevalence of chronic ulcers has been increased among elderly (e.g., pressure ulcers) [2]. The global burden of diabetes has been rising rapidly, and it is estimated that more than 425 million people suffer from diabetes all over the world, increasing to 628 million by 2045 [3]. International Diabetes Federation has estimated that 19%–34% of diabetic patients will experience a diabetic foot ulcer, and foot ulcers affect 9.1–26.1 million people with diabetes annually all over the world [4].

Reports indicate that 1–3 million people in the United States suffer from pressure ulcer annually that causes a remarkable financial burden for healthcare system [5].

According to the first comprehensive investigation of Medicare based on 2014 claims data, approximately 8.2 million people in the United States had experienced one of the wound types or infection with total spending ranged from \$28.1 to \$96.8 billion [5].

One percent of the global burden of diseases is related to burns, leading to more than 7.1 million injuries and 265,000 deaths all over the world annually [6].

Accurate wound assessment and determining the best wound care plan can significantly reduce the financial burden.

Atlas of Wound Healing. https://doi.org/10.1016/B978-0-323-67968-8.00001-X

CHAPTER 2

Wound Anatomy

A wound is an injury to the living tissue caused by accident, violence, surgery, or some chronic diseases; that is typically defined by breaking of the skin membrane and usually damage to underlying tissues or organs. Fig. 2.1 shows a wound with disruption in skin continuity.

Anatomically, a wound is defined by an external or internal breakdown in the normal continuity of Extra Cellular Matrix (ECM) and epithelium; and the loss of the protective function of the skin, with or without damage to the underlying connective tissue (i.e., vessels, nerves, muscles, or bone).

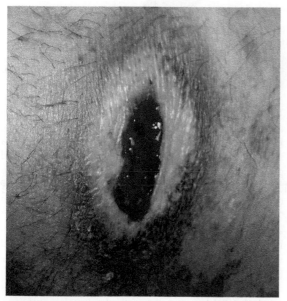

FIG. 2.1 A wound with discontinuity in skin and probably damage in underlying tissues.

Appropriate initial wound management is vital for accelerated healing and successful treatment. Therefore, understanding the anatomy and physiology of the wound-involved tissues and knowing their remodeling process are critical for effective treatment. Wound-related tissues are shown in Fig. 2.2.

WHICH TISSUES MIGHT BE DAMAGED IN WOUNDS?

There are four main types of tissue in the human body: epithelial, muscle, connective, and nervous tissues, which are made of specialized cells that are grouped together according to structure and function. Fig. 2.3 illustrates the schematic of these tissues.

Depending on the wound site and severity, any of the following tissues can be involved:

EPITHELIAL TISSUE

Epithelium, one of the four basic types of mammalian tissue, covers the outmost surfaces of organs and blood vessels, as well as, the inner surfaces of many internal organs. Epidermis, the outermost layer of normal healthy skin, is the largest epithelium of the human body.

Epithelial tissue has three main cell types: squamous (flat), columnar, and cuboidal, which can be arranged in single, double, or more layers of cells. Epithelium has many functions including protection, selective transcellular transport, and sensing [6,7].

There are no vessels in epithelial tissues; thus, the underlying connective tissues deliver the nutrition via diffusion through the cell junctions of the basement membrane.

Mostly, when an open wound occurs, the skin is damaged and loses its continuity due to the breakdown in epithelial tissue. Thus, comprehensive knowledge of structure and functions of the normal human skin is essential for understanding the wound pathophysiology.

Skin

Skin, the largest and primary protective organ in the human body, maintains a first-order physical barrier between the internal and external environments and acts as a barrier against outside pathogens and excessive loss of water or other nutrients. Generally, in direct contact with the outside environment, the skin plays a key role in immunologic surveillance, sensory perception, regulation of body temperature, and protection against trauma and UV radiation.

Atlas of Wound Healing. https://doi.org/10.1016/B978-0-323-67968-8.00002-1

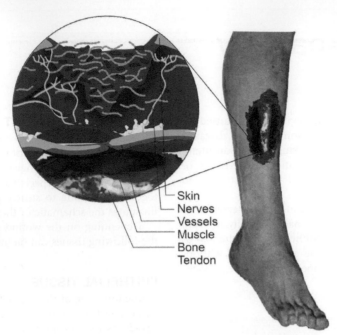

Skin
Nerves
Vessels
Muscle
Bone
Tendon

FIG. 2.2 A wound typically involves several tissues.

The skin is comprised of three layers: epidermis, dermis, and hypodermis, which are conserved across species with slight but significant differences. These well-separated layers work together to provide the multifunctional performance of skin [8–10]. Figs. 2.4 and 2.5 show functions and structure of the skin, respectively.

Epidermis

The epidermis is the external layer of the skin with a narrowed stratified structure formed by five well-defined epithelial sublayers. The major cell type in this layer is keratinocyte, which undergoes gradual differentiation from the boundary layer to the skin surface to provide an effective hierarchical barrier. The outer layer cells are dead and lose their nucleus and cytoplasm, instead of containing a tough, resistant protein called keratin that makes the epithelium waterproof. Keratinocytes are responsible for keratin synthesis, as well as the essential cytokines for wound healing. This layer protects the inner organs against UV and outside environment through melanocytes and Langerhans cells [11,12].

Dermis

The dermis, located deep in the epidermis, between the basement membrane and subcutaneous fat, houses

connective tissues, nerves, blood vessels, lymphatic vessels, hair follicles, sebaceous glands, and sweat glands.

The thickness of the dermis varies from less than 1 mm in the eyelids and over 5 mm in the back and is approximately 15–40 times thicker than the epidermis. Fibroblast is the major cell type of the dermis with a specialized ECM in two forms: fibrous proteins and ground substances.

Collagen fibers composed approximately 75% of the dry weight and 30% of the volume of the dermis with 75% collagen type I and 15% type III. The amount and quality of collagen decrease during aging. Elastin is another prominent fiber in dermis ECM, associated with the elasticity and synthesized during the fetal life by fibroblasts.

The ground substances, as a gel-like amorphous network, fill the space beneath the basal membrane, and the cells and the fibrous ECM immersed in them. The main components of ground substances are proteoglycans, glycoproteins, and hyaluronic acid that are mostly synthetized by fibroblasts [11,13]. Different cells, ECM environments, and underlying tissues of the skin sublayers are shown in Fig. 2.6.

Hypodermis

The hypodermis is the deepest layer of the skin that is responsible for attaching the dermis to muscles and

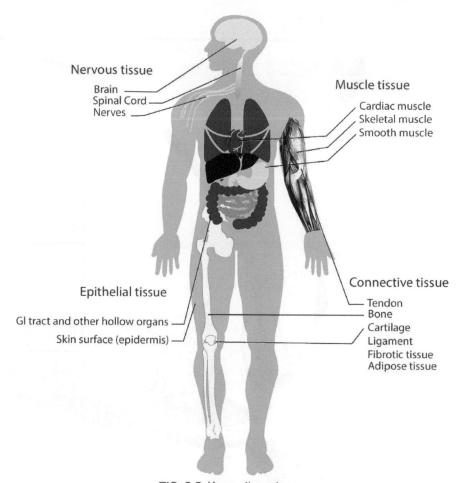

Nervous tissue
Brain
Spinal Cord
Nerves

Muscle tissue
Cardiac muscle
Skeletal muscle
Smooth muscle

Epithelial tissue
GI tract and other hollow organs
Skin surface (epidermis)

Connective tissue
Tendon
Bone
Cartilage
Ligament
Fibrotic tissue
Adipose tissue

FIG. 2.3 Human tissue types.

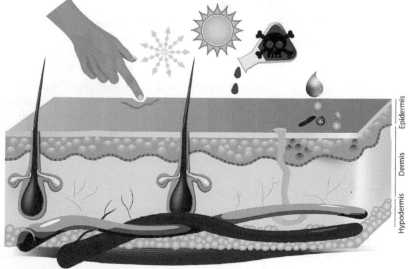

Epidermis

Dermis

Hypodermis

Function

- Appearance
- Physical barrier against the external
  environment
- Thermal regulation
- Water proof barrier preventing from
  loss of essential nutrients
- Delivery of nutrients
- Removal of waste materials and liquids
- Protection against UV
- Place for vascular networks, lymphatic
  vessels and nerves
- Providing Mechanical stability
- Sensation
- Fat storage
- Forming tight junctions
- Keeping lymphocytes in place

FIG. 2.4 Skin functions.

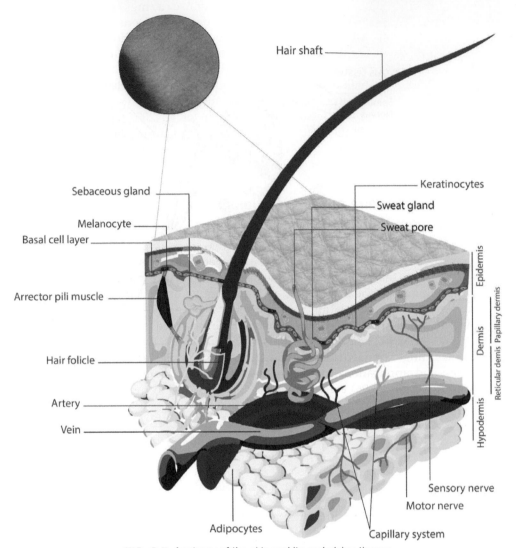

Hair shaft

Keratinocytes

Sweat gland

Sweat pore

Sebaceous gland

Melanocyte

Basal cell layer

Arrector pili muscle

Hair follicle

Artery

Vein

Epidermis

Papillary dermis

Dermis

Reticular dermis

Hypodermis

Sensory nerve

Motor nerve

Adipocytes

Capillary system

FIG. 2.5 Anatomy of the skin and its underlying tissues.

bones, houses the blood vessels and nerves, and has a key role in controlling the body temperature. The major cell type in this layer is adipocyte, and the main component is adipose tissue made of triglyceride that houses the body natural fat [10].

MUSCLES

Muscle is a soft and specialized tissue, which causes contracting and applying forces to various parts of the body. There are three types of muscle tissue: skeletal or striated muscle, smooth or nonstriated muscle, and cardiac muscle. Fibrous muscle cells, that is, myocytes,

connect together and form specialized muscle tissues in sheets (cardiac muscle) and fibers (skeletal muscles). When there is a wound, different types of muscle tissue can be injured depending on the wound depth and severity, including underlying skeletal muscle, and the striated muscular tissue of the vascular system.

Skeletal Muscle

In some wounds, the skeletal muscle tissue is partially involved. The most common injury of muscles is strain, a type of acute injury that occurs to the muscle or tendon, with a different level of severity. Skeletal

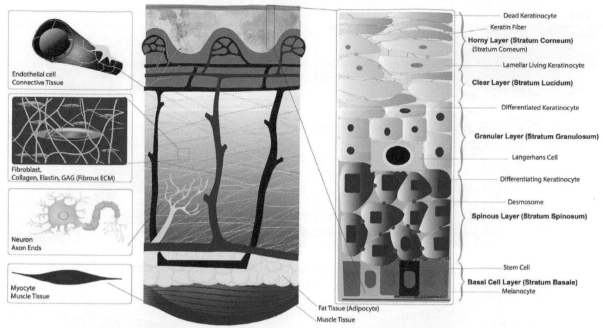

FIG. 2.6 Different cells and ECMs can be found in a wound including epidermis, dermis, hypodermis, vessel, muscle, nerve, and lymphatic vessel.

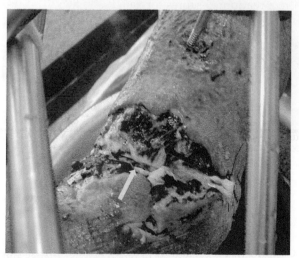

FIG. 2.7 A traumatic wound with damaged muscle (black arrow) and tendon rapture (yellow arrow).

muscles are relatively more vulnerable to acute injuries such as trauma or burn, due to their superficial location [14]. Fig. 2.7 shows a traumatic wound with injured muscle. However, the skeletal muscle can be damaged in chronic wounds due to the hypoxia and insufficient blood supply.

CONNECTIVE TISSUE

Connective tissue is characterized by a fibrous ECM, rich in collagen and elastin. This type of tissue is found everywhere in the body and contains five major cell types: fibroblasts, adipocytes, macrophages, mast cells, and endothelial cells.

When a wound occurs, skin as the most involved organ loses its integrity and its structural framework. In addition, the underlying connective tissue, that is, epidermis, adipose tissue, bone, tendon, and fascia (the fibrotic membrane that covers muscles, bones, blood vessels, and nerves) can be damaged depending on the extent of injury and the surrounding ECM loses its consistency and functions [15].

Bone

Bone is a type of dense connective tissue with a mineralized porous but rigid structure. Four types of cell can be found in the bone: osteocytes, osteoblasts, osteoclasts, and bone lining cells. Bone exerts important functions in the body, such as mobility, support, and protection of soft internal tissues, calcium and phosphate storage, and harboring of bone marrow [16].

Severe traumas or some third-degree burns can cause bone injuries or bone exposure while diabetic wounds can be diagnosed with the exposed bone and osteomyelitis, which lead to foot amputation, systemic

(A)

(C)

(B)

(D)

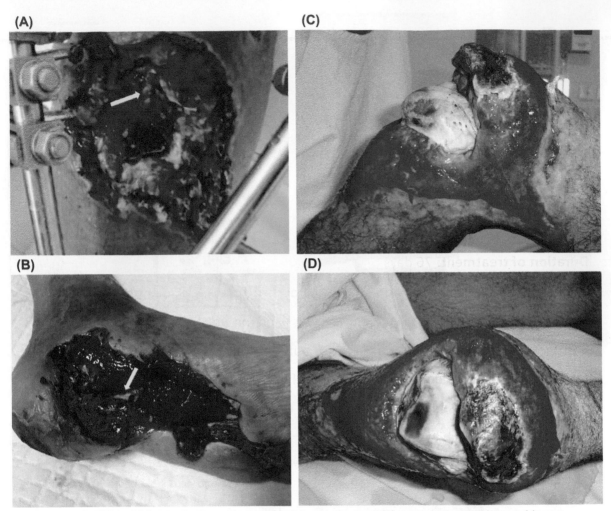

FIG. 2.8 Exposed bone can be occur in different types of wound **(A)** a traumatic wound caused by car accident **(B)** a diabetic foot ulcer **(C)** and **(D)** an infected surgical wound.

infection, and death. The exposed bone may be found in various types of wound, such as traumatic wounds, pressure ulcers, and diabetic ulcers. Fig. 2.8 shows exposed bone in an acute wound and a chronic ulcer.

Commonly, the healthy exposed bone appears in white or pale yellow. To avoid the adverse consequences of the exposed bone such as necrosis and infection, the wound surface should be moisturized to encourage the granulation tissue formation, which covers the exposed bone. If the wound does not heal, it is important to rule out osteomyelitis as a cause for impaired healing. If osteomyelitis is left without treatment, the wound closure is delayed and increases the risk of amputation or systemic infection [17].

Blood Vessels

There are two main types of blood vessels: arteries and veins, with a thick and strong wall composed of connective tissue and smooth muscle. The particular part of the vascular system associated with skin is located in the dermal deep layer to form a horizontal network consisting of two interconnected plexuses: the superficial plexus at the junction of the papillary and reticular dermis composed of postcapillary venules that supplies the dermal papillae. The deeper plexus at the dermis—hypodermis interface, which is supplied by larger blood vessels [18]. Arterial or venous disorders can cause chronic wounds called vascular ulcers.

Lymphatic Vessel

The lymphatic capillaries are extended through the postcapillary lymph vessels to the dermal and subcutaneous lymph vessels, and their structure is not regular as that of the blood vessels. The endothelial cells of the lymph capillaries are thin and are surrounded by loose collagen and elastic fibers. Lymphatic ulcers can develop because of damage to the lymphatic vessels or lymphedema [18].

NERVES

In the peripheral nervous system, a bundle of axons, that is, nerve, transmits electrochemical signals from axons to the peripheral organs. Nerve bundles with microvessels are found in neurovascular bundles of the dermis. Dermal papillae houses Meissner corpuscles, which enable touch in the hands and feet [18].

Generally, there are three types of nerves: (1) Motor nerves send impulses from brain and spinal cord to muscles. (2) The sensory nerves transmit tactile, pressure, pain, and temperature sensation. (3) The autonomic nerves are responsible for the function of blood vessels and sweat glands [13]. In uncontrolled diabetes, autonomic neuropathy destroys the sympathetic component of the autonomic nervous system that controls vasoconstriction in peripheral blood vessels [19,20].

Depending on the extent of injury, axons and surrounding connective tissues in nerves can be damaged. The most severe repairable injury occurs in third degree wounds, where the axons and inner layer of connective tissue (endoneurium) are damaged while the outer thicker layers (perineurium and epineurium) remain intact. In more severe damages where the entire connective tissue is disrupted, fibroblasts fill the damaged site by fibrous ECM that prevents the cut axon from regenerating and connecting to the original nerve cell [21].

CHAPTER 3

Wound Healing Process

Wound healing is a complex and dynamic process in which dead cells, damaged Extra Cellular Matrix (ECM), missing structures, and devitalized tissues are replaced by new cells and tissues. As an immediate response to tissue damage, wound healing involves a large number of biochemical and cellular processes.

WOUND HEALING PHASES

The wound healing process can be divided into four separated, but overlapping phases: hemostasis, inflammation, proliferation, and remodeling. Fig. 3.1 shows these phases against time.

Hemostasis

A breakdown in tissue integrity following injury causes bleeding, which fills the wound and exposes the blood to various components of the ECM. After platelets aggregation, factor XII is activated, thereby forming fibrin clot, which leads to hemostasis. The fibrin clot acts as a preliminary matrix within the wound space into which cells can migrate. After the fibrin clot forms, another mechanism is activated, that is, fibrinolysis, which prevents clot extension and dissolves the fibrin clot to provide space for further cell migration and proceeds to the next stage of healing (Fig. 3.2).

Inflammation

The inflammatory phase begins immediately after tissue injury. During this phase, the fibrin clot degrades and the capillaries dilate and become permeable, releasing plasma and main inflammatory cell (i.e., neutrophils and macrophages) into the injury site and activating the complement system. Neutrophils recruit to the wound immediately after injury and reach their maximum within 24–48 h. In fact, they are the first line of defense against infection, and their main function is to phagocyte debris and pathogens. During the digestion, neutrophils die and release intracellular enzymes, which further digest the tissue. As fibrin is broken down, the degradation products attract fibroblasts and epithelial cells (Fig. 3.2).

Approximately 2 or 3 days after injury, blood monocytes release tissue macrophages, which also destroy bacteria and debris through phagocytosis. The other function of macrophages is to release biological regulators, including cytokines, growth factors, and proteolytic enzymes, which are necessary for the normal

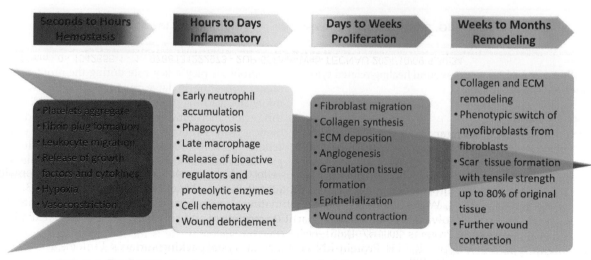

FIG. 3.1 The four phases of wound healing (hemostasis, inflammatory, proliferative, and remodeling).

Atlas of Wound Healing. https://doi.org/10.1016/B978-0-323-67968-8.00003-3

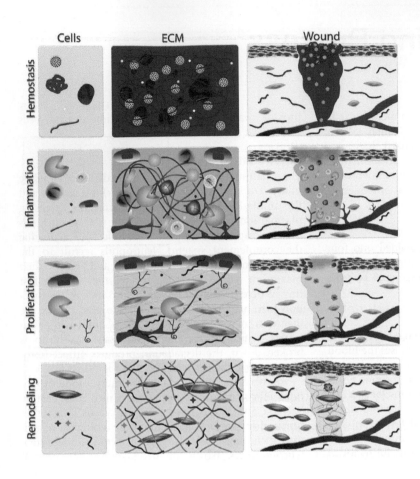

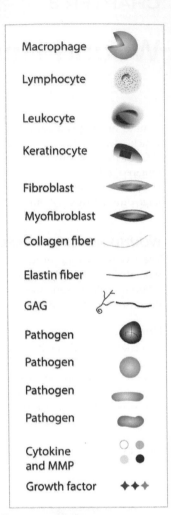

FIG. 3.2 Wound healing phases: main cell types, ECM, and tissues.

healing process [22]. Major wound healing-related cytokines are shown in Table 3.1.

Proliferation

The proliferation phase approximately begins from day 4 to day 21 after injury. This phase is characterized by granulation tissue formation in the wound space and keratinocytes migration to regenerate epithelial tissue and restore the epidermis layer continuity.

During this phase, the new tissue forms by a matrix of collagen, elastin, and glycosaminoglycans (GAGs), and other fibrous proteins, and is filled by fibrin and fibronectin. Fibroblasts move into the wound space and proliferate to synthetize more collagen fibers (Fig. 3.2).

Fibroblasts play a key role during the proliferation phase, appearing in large numbers within 3 days of injury and reaching peak levels on the 7th day. During this period, they undergo intense proliferative and synthetic activity. Fibroblasts synthesize and deposit extracellular proteins during wound healing, producing growth factors and angiogenic factors that regulate cell proliferation and angiogenesis [22]. The main cytokines of this phase are shown in Table 3.1.

Remodeling

The remodeling phase is the longest phase of wound healing and takes time from 21 days to 1 year. Remodeling is characterized by collagen rearrangement and wound contraction.

TABLE 3.1
Cytokines Role in Wound Healing [22, 23]

Cytokine	Cell Source	Effect on Wound Healing
Platelet derived growth factor (PDGF)	Platelets, Keratinocytes, Macrophages, Endothelial cells, Fibroblasts	• Inflammation • Collagen and protein synthesis • Granulation tissue formation • Reepithelialization • Matrix formation • Remodeling
Transforming growth factor α (TGF-α)	Epithelial cells, Macrophages, Platelets, Endothelial cells	• Chemotaxis • Epithelialization
Transforming growth factor β (TGF-β)	Epithelial cells, Macrophages, Platelets, Neutrophils, Keratinocytes, Lymphocytes, Fibroblasts	• Inflammation • Granulation tissue formation • Reepithelialization • Matrix formation • Remodeling
Fibroblast growth factor (FGF)	Macrophages, Fibroblasts, Endothelial cells, Keratinocytes, Mast Cells, Smooth muscle cells Chondrocytes	• Angiogenesis • Granulation tissue formation • Reepithelialization • Matrix formation • Remodeling
Epidermal growth factor (EGF)	Keratinocytes, Fibroblasts, Platelets, Macrophages	• Neovascularization • Reepithelialization
Insulin-like growth factor (IGF)	Liver, Skeletal muscle	• Keratinocyte and fibroblast proliferation • Angiogenesis
Vascular Endothelial Growth Factor (VEGF)	Platelets, Neutrophils, Macrophages, Endothelial cells, Smooth muscle cells, Fibroblasts	• Granulation tissue formation
Interleukin-1 (IL-1)	Neutrophils, Monocytes, Macrophages, Keratinocytes	• Inflammation • Reepithelialization
Interleukin-1 (IL-6)	Neutrophils, Macrophages	• Inflammation • Reepithelialization
Tumor Necrosis Factor TNF-α	Neutrophils, Macrophages	• Inflammation • Reepithelialization
Interferon	T-cells, Natural killer (NK)	• Macrophages

When the rate of collagen synthesis and degradation equalize, the remodeling phase of tissue healing begins [20]. During this phase, collagen type I is changed to collagen type III, and the newly synthesized collagen fibers are rearranged, cross-linked, and aligned along mechanical tension lines. The duration of this phase is ranging from 3 to 21 days and it depends on the wound size, severity and closure type.

In this phase, collagen gains approximately 20% of its initial tensile strength by the third week, and reaches 80% after 12 weeks. The maximum tensile strength of scar tissue is approximately 80% of that of normal healthy skin (Fig. 3.2).

Mostly, the wound healing phases progress in a predictable, timely manner; otherwise, the healing may stop or progress inadequately leading to chronic wound or pathological scar formation.

IMPORTANT PARAMETERS FOR SUCCESSFUL WOUND HEALING

ECM Proteins

ECM consists of proteins and polysaccharides called proteoglycans, glycoproteins, and GAGs. The two main classes of matrix proteins are fibrous proteins (collagen, elastin, and fibronectin). Collagen is the most abundant protein in mammals and accounts for 70%–80% of the dry weight of the dermis and is mostly synthetized by fibroblasts.

Elastin is responsible for tissue elasticity and resilience. It is composed of fibrous coils that stretch and return to their original form and helps to maintain tissue shape. Elastin represents only 2%–4% of the human skin's dry weight.

Fibronectin is a fibrous molecule that provides anchors for cell adhesion and is responsible for cell–cell or cell–ECM interactions. It has a key role in the remodeling phase, acting as a mediator for physical interactions between cells and deposited collagen fibers, providing a preliminary matrix.

Proteoglycans consist of a protein backbone branched with a number of polysaccharide side chains in several types, while the glyco proteins are composed of a polysaccharide backbone with amino acid side chains. GAG chains are long unbranched polysaccharides with amino-sugars repeating disaccharides. Proteoglycans are characterized by their diverse structural and organizational functions in tissue and a highly hydrated gel-like ground substance, with up to 95% (w/w) carbohydrates.

Angiogenesis Process

As one of the key parts of wound healing, angiogenesis is a dynamic process through which new vessels are formed to carry blood for nutrients and oxygen delivery. The vascular endothelial cells arise from the end of damaged vessels and capillaries, present at the wound edges, and form new capillaries. These capillaries continue growing to meet the other growing capillaries and connect with each other to form a capillary network and allow blood circulation.

Epithelialization Process

Epithelial healing, or epithelialization, which begins a few hours after injury, is another important feature of healing. Marginal basal cells, which are normally firmly attached to the underlying dermis, change their cell adhesion behavior and start to detach, migrating in a train fashion across the provisional matrix. This horizontal movement is stopped when cells meet.

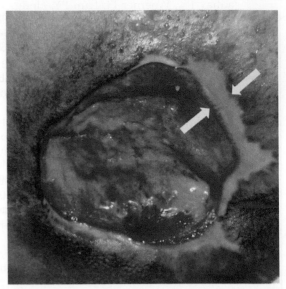

FIG. 3.3 Yellow arrows indicate the epithelial tissue that appears from the wound edge.

In epithelial tissue, keratinocytes travel from the edges of the wound, and slowly grow over the granulating tissue with deep pink color that eventually turns into light purple. A large amount of epithelizing tissue is usually an indicator of successful wound healing [3]. Fig. 3.3 shows the new epithelial tissue formation.

Wound Contraction

The final sign of the proliferation phase is wound contraction, which normally starts 5 days after injury. Wound contraction is a dynamic process through which connective tissue matrix is formed by collagen fibers synthetized by newly migrated fibroblasts. Then, fibroblasts differentiate to myofibroblasts that are responsible for tensile force to pull the wound edges toward the wound center, which results in gradually reducing the wound area (Fig. 3.4). Wound contraction decreases the healing time by inhibiting the oversynthesis of ECM proteins. The contractile activity of fibroblasts and myofibroblasts provides the force for the contraction [3, 22, 24].

Matrix Metalloproteinases

Proteases, especially the matrix metalloproteinases (MMPs), play key roles in all phases of normal wound healing (see Table 3.2). During the inflammatory phase, damaged extracellular matrix proteins, particularly collagen fibers, are degraded by MMPs to align the newly synthesized collagen fibers, correctly, which

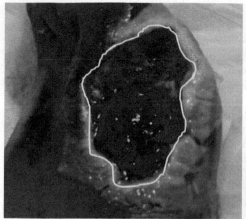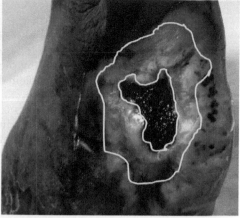

FIG. 3.4 Wound contraction.

TABLE 3.2
The Role of MMP Family in Wound Healing [25, 26]

	MMPs	Substrates	Cell Source	Role in Wound Healing
Collagenases	MMP-1 collagenase-1	Collagen I, II, III, VII, and X; aggrecan; serpins; alpha2-macroglobulin; kallikrein; chymase	• Proliferating and migrating keratinocytes • Fibroblasts	• Promotes human keratinocyte migration on fibrillar collagen • Expressed by keratinocytes at their trailing membrane edge during wound healing • Overexpression in keratinocytes delays reepithelialization
	MMP-8 collagenase-2	Collagen I, II, and III; aggrecan; serpins; 2-MG	• Neutrophils	• Cleaves collagens, predominant collagenase in healing wounds
	MMP-13 collagenase-3	Collagen I, II, III, IV, IX, X, and XIV; gelatin; fibronectin; laminin; tenascin; aggrecan; fibrillin; serpins	• Fibroblasts	• Promotes reepithelialization indirectly by affecting wound contraction
Gelatinases	MMP-2* gelatinase A	Gelatin; collagen I, IV, V, VII, and X; laminin; aggrecan; fibronectin; tenascin	• Fibroblasts	• Accelerates cell migration
	MMP-9* gelatinase B	Gelatin; collagens I, III, IV, V, and VII; aggrecan; elastin; fibrillin	• Keratinocytes • Neutrophils • Macrophages • Endothelial cells	• Expressed by keratinocytes at the leading edge of the wound • Promotes cell migration and reepithelialization except in cornea

Continued

TABLE 3.2
The Role of MMP Family in Wound Healing [25, 26]—cont'd

	MMPs	Substrates	Cell Source	Role in Wound Healing
Stromelysins	MMP-3 stromelysin-1	Collagen IV, V, IX, and X; fibronectin; elastin; gelatin; aggrecan; nidogen; fibrillin; E-cadherin	• Basal proliferating keratinocytes • Fibroblasts	• Expressed by keratinocytes at the proximal proliferating population that supplies the leading edge during wound healing • Affects wound contraction
	MMP-10 stromelysin-2	Collagen IV, V, IX, and X; fibronectin; elastin; gelatin; laminin; aggrecan, nidogen; E-cadherin	• Migrating keratinocyte • Fibroblasts	• Expressed by keratinocytes at the leading edge of the wound
Matrilysins	MMP-7 matrilysin	Elastin; fibronectin; laminin; nidogen; collagen IV; tenascin; versican; 1-proteinase inhibitor; E-cadherin; tumor necrosis factor		• Required for reepithelialization of mucosal wounds
Metalloelastases	MMP-12 metalloeslastase	Collagen IV; gelatin; fibronectin; laminin; vitronectin; elastin; fibrillin; 1-proteinase inhibitor; apolipoprotein A	• Macrophages	• Macrophage specific (not expressed by epithelial cells)
Membrane-type MMPs	MMP-14 MT1-MMP	Collagen I, II, and III; gelatin; fibronectin; laminin; vitronectin; aggrecan; tenascin; nidogen; perlecan; fibrillin; 1-proteinase inhibitor; alpha2-macroglobulin; fibrin	• Migrating keratinocytes	• Promotes keratinocyte outgrowth, airway reepithelialization and cell migration

*MMP-2 and MMP-9 have been found in elevated amounts in infected wounds.

enable the fibroblasts migration. To degrade the damaged collagens, collagenase divides the collagen fibers into two parts, and then gelatinase cuts it down into smaller fragments for further phagocytosis by neutrophils and macrophages.

MMPs have a significant role in angiogenesis by endothelial cells detachment through removing the endothelial basement membrane, which enables the new capillary network formation. Furthermore, MMPs are essential for wound contraction to shape the newly formed ECM correctly, based on the surrounding connective tissue pattern.

The actions of MMPs are controlled by the tissue inhibitors of metalloproteinases (TIMPs), that is, their natural inhibitors [3, 22].

MMPs along with their inhibitors play an essential role in reepithelialization by regulating ECM degradation and deposition. MMP inhibitors (MMPI) can be both endogenous and exogenous. TIMPs including four different subtypes (TIMP-1, TIMP-2, TIMP-3, and TIMP-4), which inhibit MMPs, are endogenous. They regulate the MMPs activity through the interaction of the N-terminal domain of the TIMP molecules and the active site of the MMP [1].

WOUND TISSUE TYPES
Devitalized Wound Tissues
Necrotic tissue
Necrotic tissue is a mass of devitalized tissue in a wound that is separated from the surrounding living tissue as a potential medium for bacterial growth. This type of tissue often sticks to the wound bed and cannot be simply removed. There are two significant types of necrotic tissue occurring in wounds: Eschar and slough.

Eschar tissue
Eschar tissue is usually dry and thick with white/black appearance [3] (Figs. 3.5 and 3.6).

Slough tissue
Slough tissue presents yellow, tan, green, or brown tissue, moist in appearance [3] (Fig. 3.7).

Scab layer
Usually after 24 h of injury on skin, clots containing platelets, fibrin, and erythrocytes will be dehydrated and form a rusty brown, dry layer called scab on wound preventing further blood loss and further dehydration of the healing skin underneath, protecting the wound, and providing a scaffold for tissue regeneration. This layer will trap pathogens; subsequently, the risk of infection will be reduced and wound healing will be impaired. By removing scabs before the usual time, red and oozing skin will be revealed and new scabs

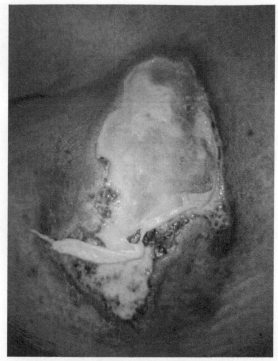

FIG. 3.6 Necrotic tissue: White eschar.

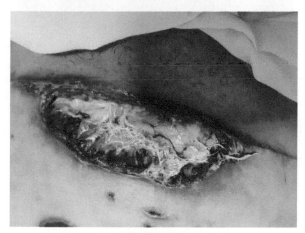

FIG. 3.7 Slough tissue.

will reform but it may lead to scar tissue formation [3] (Fig. 3.8).

Callus tissue
As a response to repeated friction, pressure, or other irritations, a thickened and hard skin called Callus tissue will appear [3] (Fig. 3.9).

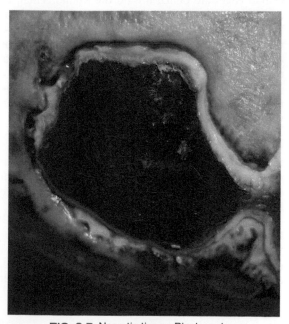

FIG. 3.5 Necrotic tissue: Black eschar.

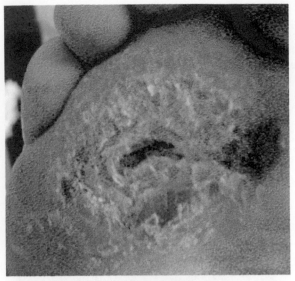

FIG. 3.8 Scab layer.

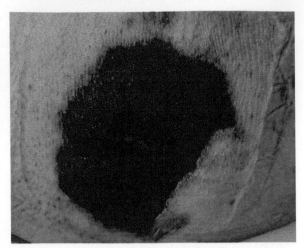

FIG. 3.10 Granulation tissue.

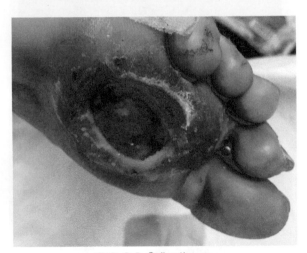

FIG. 3.9 Callus tissue.

Regenerating Wound Tissues
Granulation tissue

Granulation tissue is formed by new connective tissue and microvessels, which are the main vehicles for delivering oxygen and nutrient during the healing process. Granulation tissue is generally characterized by a rough and moist surface, and it is pink or light red in color.

Granulation tissue provides the foundation for epithelial tissue to grow and cover the wound surface [3] (Fig. 3.10).

New epithelial tissue

New epithelial tissue forms during the epidermal regeneration by basal keratinocytes migration to the wound surface. They cover the wound surface by proliferating from wound edges to the center. Epithelial tissue often appears deep pink in color (Fig. 3.3).

TYPES OF WOUND CLOSURE

Wound healing is a dynamic process through which the wound edges are pulled toward the wound center, to close the wound by tissue regeneration. Wounds heal by different intentions depending on whether the wound closure is performed by stitching or left without any intervention to repair the damaged tissue by its own.

There are three types of wound healing to describe the various ways for full-thickness wound healing with surgical wounds as the reference point:

Primary Wound Healing

Wounds that heal through primary intention mainly do not involve the loss of tissue, for example, superficial traumatic wounds or surgical wounds, and first-degree burn.

Secondary Wound Healing

Wounds involve some degree of tissue loss, for example, pressure ulcers, burns, wound dehiscence, and traumatic injuries. They take longer to heal, result in scarring, and have a higher rate of complications.

Tertiary Wound Healing

These wounds, also known as delayed primary closure, are left open for several days to allow treatment of edema, infection, or exudate drainage. They are usually closed with sutures or some other skin closure techniques.

The schematic of wound healing types are shown in Fig. 3.11.

FACTORS THAT IMPAIR WOUND HEALING

As mentioned earlier, all four phases of wound healing must occur in the appropriate time and sequence to have a normal successful wound healing process. However, these phases can be interfered by one or more phases, which result in impaired wound healing. These factors can be categorized into two classes. Table 3.3 shows these factors.

Age

According to the WHO report on aging and health, the world's population is aging rapidly and life expectancy is reported approximately more than 60 [27]. As a serious global health issue, aging affects the normal physiological state and causes age-related disease, which involves most elderly people. For example, aging is one of the main risk factors for impaired wound healing and chronic ulcer formation. Different phases of wound healing can be influenced by aging:

1. Hemostasis phase: Increasing the platelet aggregation and degranulation
2. Inflammatory phase: Early increase in neutrophils, delayed monocyte infiltration, and macrophage functions

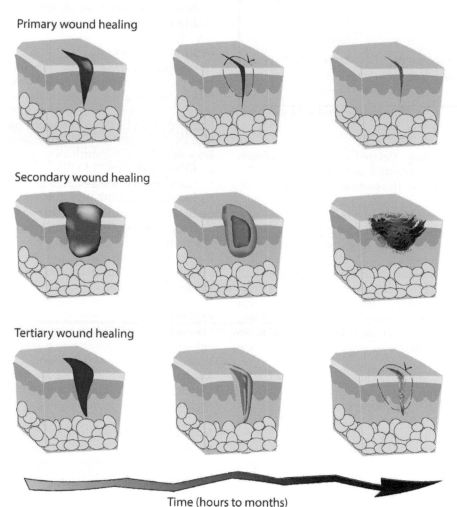

Primary wound healing

Secondary wound healing

Tertiary wound healing

Time (hours to months)

FIG. 3.11 Types of wound healing.

TABLE 3.3
Factors Affect Wound Healing

General Factors	Local Factor
Age	Inadequate blood supply
Immobility	Increased skin tension
Obesity	Poor surgical opposition
Smoking or other addictions	Wound dehiscence
Shock of any cause	Poor venous drainage
Malnutrition	Prescience of foreign body
Chronic disease	Moisture level
Systemic malignancy and terminal illness	Wound temperature
Chemotherapy	Infection
Radiotherapy	Biofilm
Immunosuppressive drugs	Excess local mobility
Inherited neutrophil disorder	Necrotic tissue formation

3. Proliferation phase: Delayed angiogenesis, collagen deposition, and reepithelialization
4. Remodeling phase: Increased scarring [28].

Life Style

Life style as a general term, including smoking habit, alcohol intake, nutrition, exercise, and stress, has major effects on wound healing.

Nicotine, an alkaloid toxic substance, impedes all phases of wound healing results in slower wound closure. Smoking impairs leukocyte activity, reduces bactericidal response of macrophages and neutrophils, decreases fibroblast migration, reduces epithelial tissue regeneration, and delays or stops wound contraction [29, 30].

Alcohol intake impairs wound healing by increasing blood glucose level and insulin resistance, which impairs inflammatory response, wound closure, angiogenesis, and collagen synthesis, as well as, imbalanced proteases [29].

Nutritional status of a patient suffering from a wound has been recognized as a key factor affecting wound healing. Nutrition deficiencies impede the normal process of wound healing. Insufficient protein causes impairment of angiogenesis, fibroblast proliferation, protein synthesis, and wound remodeling. People with low socioeconomic status, elderly patients, patients with chronic ulcers, diabetes, and malabsorption issues are at high risk of malnutrition [30, 31].

Studies have demonstrated that psychological stress is also a cause of significant delay in wound healing by upregulating glucocorticoids (GCs), reduction of proinflammatory cytokines IL-1β, IL-6, TNF-α, and decreasing expression of IL-1α and IL-8 at wound sites, in human and animals [30].

Physical training is a low-cost clinically intervention to speed up wound healing. Many researches revealed that exercise accelerates wound healing in human and animals, especially in venous ulcers and diabetic foot ulcers. Exercise decreases the level of inflammatory markers in the blood, which results in faster wound healing [32−36].

Systemic Diseases

Uncontrolled diabetes causes abnormality in cellular functions that impede all phases of wound healing in patients suffering from acute or chronic wounds (e.g., surgical incisions, pressure ulcers, etc.) [29]. The impaired wound healing in diabetic patients is due to hypoxia, neuropathy, inadequate angiogenesis, high amounts of metalloproteinases, and insufficient immune response [30].

Other systemic diseases, such as cancer, cardiovascular disorders, kidney failure, high blood pressure, and metabolic disorders can delay the wound healing process, significantly. On the other hand, the therapeutic approach for mentioned diseases might interrupt wound healing or lead to new ulcer formation, for example, ulcers caused by chemotherapy and radiotherapy [37].

Maceration

Maceration is characterized by a softening and whitening swollen skin, which breaks down the skin's integrity and results in wound enlargement. Poor control of wound exudate, prolonged exposure to moisture, inappropriate dressing, or excessive perspiration of urine can lead to maceration in surrounding skin (Fig. 3.12) [38].

Necrotic Tissue

Necrotic tissue as a devitalized tissue can delay wound healing due to inability to regenerate. It must be removed before treatment through debridement process.

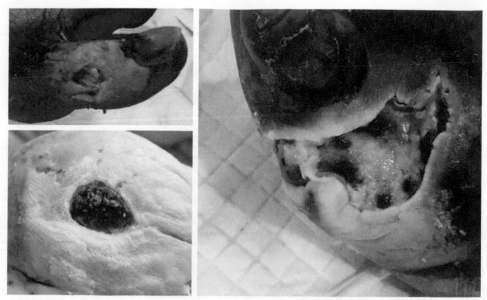

FIG. 3.12 Macerated wound tissue.

Infection

Normally pathogens are present on the skin surface, and enter into the underlying tissues, once a wound is occured. The pathogens population and replication rate determine the wound infection status as contamination, colonization, localized infection, and invasive infection. Pathogens cause an interruption in the immune response before inflammatory phase and impede wound healing.

An infected wound is characterized by exudate, induration, erythema, and/or fever. Culturing the wound identifies the intensity and type of pathogens, for that the appropriate antibiotic therapy can be prescribed. In case of bone exposure in pressure ulcers, diabetic foot ulcers, or full thickness wounds, the patient should be examined for signs of osteomyelitis [30, 38].

Wound Biofilm

Adverse microorganisms can be attached to the wound surface and embedded into a self-producing matrix of extracellular polymeric substances (EPS), known as biofilm, which is composed of polysaccharides, proteins, lipids, genetic materials, and microbial cells. Biofilm provides a well-shaped 3D environment for the growth and differentiation of microbial cells, which results in biofilm establishment and adverse genetic development through RNA/DNA exchange. Fig. 3.13 shows the schematic of biofilms formed on the surface of a chronic wound.

Biofilms significantly impair wound healing, particularly in chronic ulcers, since biofilms act as an impermeable, protective, slimy barrier, which is firmly attached to the wound surface.

Biofilms trigger a chronic inflammatory response that results in the accumulation of neutrophils and macrophages around biofilm. These inflammatory cells secrete high amounts of reactive oxygen species, which dissolve biofilm and affect the surrounding tissue, adversely. To detach biofilm from the wound surface, neutrophils and macrophages release high amounts of MMPs, which cause a prolonged inflammatory response and impaired wound healing process.

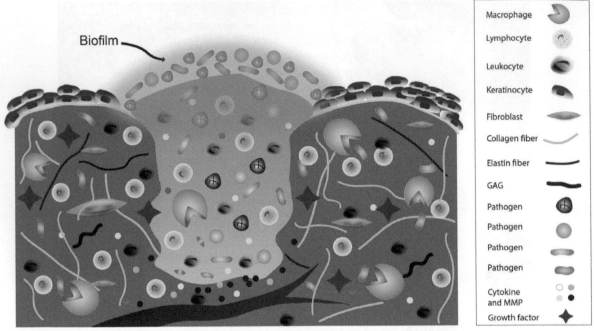

FIG. 3.13 Wound biofilm is an impermeable layer on the wound surface.

CHAPTER 4

Wound Assessment

Before starting the main procedure of wound assessment, a preassessment must be performed as follows:

- Wound cause
- Wound duration
- Risk of death

To prescribe an effective treatment and schedule a suitable wound care plan, it is necessary to assess the wound in different aspects. In fact, wound assessment along with patient's medical history can extremely influence the treatment quality and duration. The wound should be examined in size, color and other characteristics. Different parts of the wound and key assessment parameters are shown in Figs. 4.1 and 4.2, respectively.

WOUND SITE

The anatomic location of the wound (i.e., left medial malleolus) should be documented (Fig. 4.3).

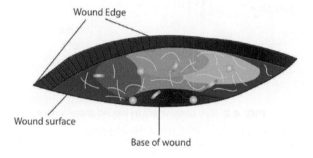

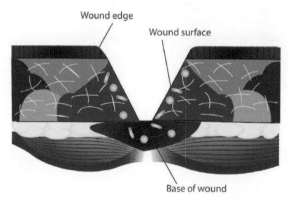

FIG. 4.1 Different parts of the wound.

Atlas of Wound Healing, https://doi.org/10.1016/B978-0-323-67968-8.00004-5

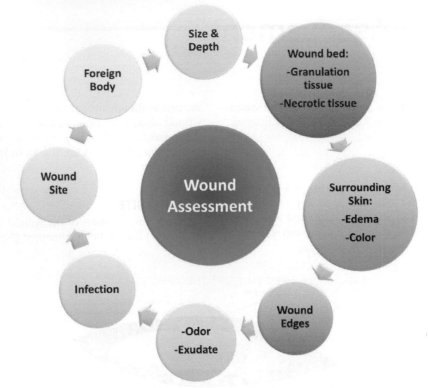

FIG. 4.2 Key parameters in wound assessment.

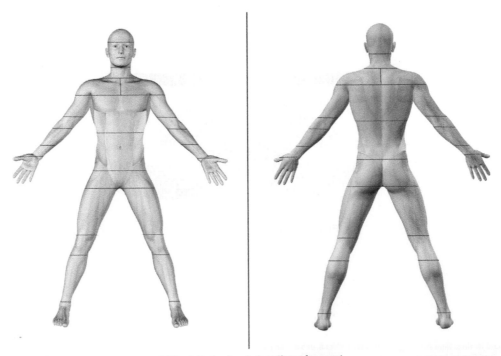

FIG. 4.3 Anatomic location of wound.

SIZE

Wound size is a high priority parameter, which is measured at the first presentation to determine the amount of tissue loss. Constant or progressive wound size during treatment, is a sign of delayed wound healing. The wound's length, width, and depth should be measured appropriately (Figs. 4.4—4.6).

DEPTH

Wound depth is another significant parameter that helps to determine the wound grading (Fig. 4.6).

WOUND BED

Proper identification of wound bed tissues specifies the wound status that will lead to appropriate treatment. As mentioned earlier, several tissue types can be found in the wound bed, such as necrotic, slough, granulation, and epithelialization tissue (Figs. 3.7 and 3.10).

WOUND EDGES

Observation and examination of wound edges can provide important information about its etiology and status (Tables 4.1 and 4.2).

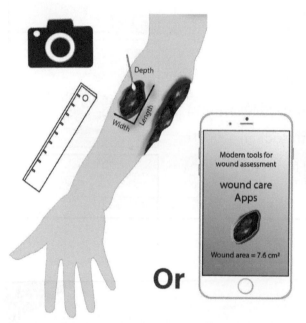

FIG. 4.4 Schematic of wound size measurement in three dimensions.

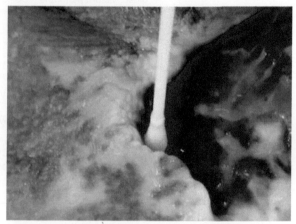

FIG. 4.6 Placing the tip of a swab in the deepest part of the wound, and marking the skin level to measure the depth of the wound.

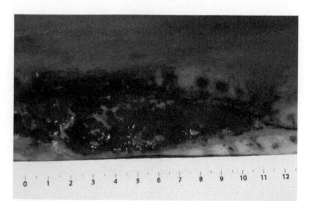

FIG. 4.5 Measuring the length of wound by a paper ruler.

TABLE 4.1
Examination of Wound Edges [20]

Sign	Causes
Red, hot skin; tenderness; and induration	Inflammation due to infection or excess pressure
Maceration (white skin)	Excess moisture due to excess wound discharge or inappropriate dressing
Rolled skin edges	Very dry wound bed
Undermining or ecchymosis of surrounding skin (loose or bruised skin edges)	Excess shearing force to the area

TABLE 4.2
Wound Edge Characteristics [39–41]

Type of Edges	More Frequent Type of Ulcer	Shape of Edges
Smooth	Surgical incision	
Irregular	Laceration, abrasion, after hydrolytic debridement	
Flat sloping	Venous ulcer	
Punched-out	Neuropathic-Arterial or vasculitic ulcer, Malum perforans (trophic ulcer)	
Rolled	Basal cell carcinoma	
Everted	Squamous cell carcinoma, poor suturing of surgical incision	
Undermining	Pressure ulcers, tuberculosis, syphilis	
Purple	Vasculitic, pyoderma gangrenosum	

SURROUNDING SKIN

By observing the skin around the wound, any change in color, temperature, and texture should be noted. An erythema or increased temperature of surrounding skin may indicate underlying infection. Fig. 4.7 shows the changes in surrounding skin following infection.

WOUND EXUDATE

Determination of a proper treatment is highly dependent on exudate levels. Thus, observation and examination of exudate is one of the significant aspects of wound assessment (Fig. 4.3). There are several types of exudates:

- Serous: clear, thin, and watery
- Sanguineous: thin red, with fresh blood
- Serosanguineous: thin, light red, and watery
- Purulent: thick, white, yellow, green, and creamy (Fig. 4.8)

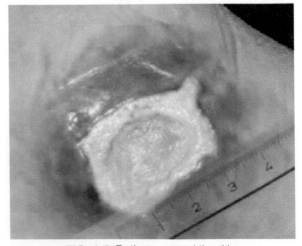

FIG. 4.7 Erythema around the skin.

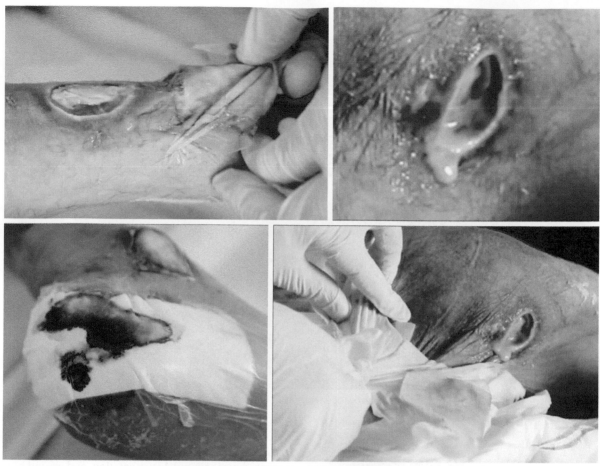

FIG. 4.8 Different types of wound exudate.

TUNNELING

Tunneling (sinus tract) is a narrow channel which could extend into any direction from the wound through the soft tissue which can lead to dead space and abscess formation (Fig. 4.9).

UNDERMINING

When the underlying wound margins is destructed, undermining occurs. It may extend in one or more directions under the wound edges (Fig. 4.10).

MODERN ASSESSMENT TOOLS

In recent years, wound assessment tools have developed and there seem to be quantitative methods for measuring the wound area, which are replacing traditional wound assessment methods. These modern tools are working based on artificial intelligence through mobile apps or computer software.

Since the introduction of smartphones, they have played a key role in various fields, including wound care. Advances in apps development and mobile hardware facilitate access to patients' records and quantitative results for wound care professionals. In addition, these fast-growing technologies are assisting the clinicians and nurses for more quality diagnosis and treatment, as a result of providing highly reliable and accurate data. On the other hand, these modern tools can be employed for educational purposes and rapid transfer of wound care knowledge, due to their interactive nature and user-friendly interface.

Currently, more than 80 various wound care apps can be found in the app market, and several recent reports have discussed the use of mobile apps for different

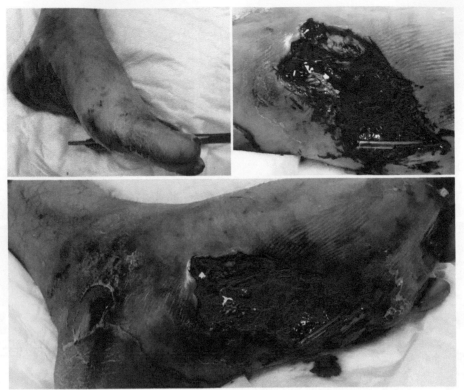

FIG. 4.9 Tunneling is a narrow opening, which has extended through the soft tissue.

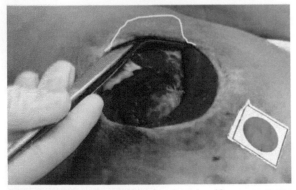

FIG. 4.10 Wound undermining may extend in one or many directions underneath the wound edges.

wound care purposes, including wound area measurement, chronic wound documentation, and wound healing monitoring through artificial intelligence, image processing techniques, and concepts of Electronic Health Records [42,43].

HEALAPP

HealApp, a mobile application developed by ChitoTech Inc., can provide continuous wound monitoring at hospitals, wound care centers, and patients' home, allowing clinicians to do follow-up care remotely with accurate information.

HealApp uses artificial intelligence to evaluate the size, topology, shape, and color of the wound and tracks the wound changes (Figs. 4.11—4.13).

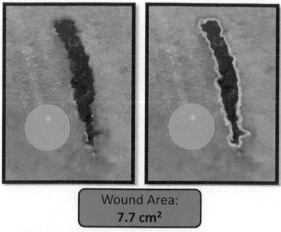

Wound Area:
7.7 cm²

FIG. 4.11 HealApp measures the wound area by drawing wound boundaries and measuring the area using a paper tag as 2D scale.

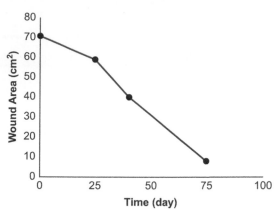

FIG. 4.13 Wound healing progression against time.

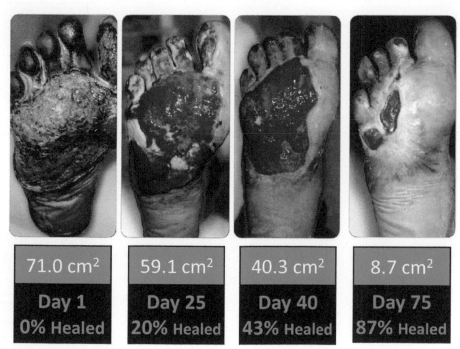

71.0 cm²	59.1 cm²	40.3 cm²	8.7 cm²
Day 1	Day 25	Day 40	Day 75
0% Healed	20% Healed	43% Healed	87% Healed

FIG. 4.12 HealApp measures the wound area and reports the area quantitatively.

CHAPTER 5

Wound Care Management

Wound care, especially chronic wound, is a major challenging issue for medical care professionals; hence, wound care management has a key role in the quality and duration of wound treatment.

Wound care management is a general term, which includes wound assessment, cleansing, appropriate treatment approach, and scar tissue management. Each of these items significantly influences the patient's quality of life and has a vital contribution in treatment outcome and costs.

Fig. 5.1 shows the different parts of wound care management.

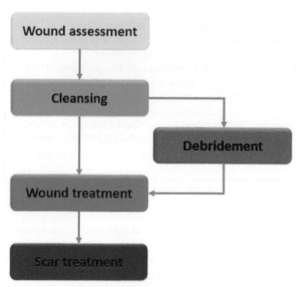

FIG. 5.1 Different parts of wound care management.

WOUND CLEANSING AND DISINFECTING

Wound cleansing is an integral part of wound management and defined by removing wound surface contaminants, foreign bodies, debris, and previous dressing residues without damaging the healthy tissues. Wound cleansing is usually performed by fluids such as normal saline or advanced antiseptics.

Antiseptics

Antiseptics are disinfectant solutions with antimicrobial effect on either intact skin or open wounds to kill or inactivate microorganisms. Some of them are effective on a broad range of pathogens, while the others are effective against one or two microbial targets. Despite the therapeutic effect of antiseptics, some of them may cause serious harmful effects on healthy and granulating tissue [44]. Table 5.1 discusses the effectiveness and limitations of several topical antiseptic solutions.

Silver Nano Colloidal Solutions

Nowadays, silver nanoparticles are known as a viable alternative to traditional antibacterial disinfectants and present a high efficiency solution for bacterial resistance. Silver had been used as an antiseptic agent from ancient era. In the past few years, considerable research has been conducted to prove the antiseptic and antimicrobial effect of silver against gram-positive and gram-negative bacteria, as well as, to its incredibly low cytotoxicity. In recent years, silver nanoparticles became a new class of antimicrobial agents, which represents a powerful approach against a wide range of pathogens.

From a structural point of view, silver nanoparticles with an extremely high aspect ratio exhibit the extraordinary physical, chemical, and biological properties. Practically, the bactericidal effectiveness of silver nanoparticles is strongly size depended, and smaller particle (<30 nm) showed an optimized antimicrobial effect. Silver nano colloidal solution is a stable colloid of silver nanoparticle, which can deliver these nanoparticles directly to the wound site.

Several mechanisms of action have been proposed for silver antibacterial effectiveness as follows:
1. Irreversible damage on bacterial cells wall and cytoplasm destruction
2. Alteration of membrane permeability and membrane damage
3. Alteration of microorganism respiration and intracellular ATP levels
4. Inhibition of DNA replication [46,47]

Atlas of Wound Healing. https://doi.org/10.1016/B978-0-323-67968-8.00005-7

TABLE 5.1
Topical Antiseptic Products Based on Chemical Origin [20,44,45]

Solution	Description	Uses	Contraindications
Normal saline	Isotonic solution without antibacterial effect	Regular wound irrigation	Dirty wounds and necrotic wounds
Hydrogen peroxide	A topical antiseptic causes vasodilation and reduces inflammation but damages healthy and granulating tissues due to cytotoxicity	Wound disinfectant suitable for mechanical debridement	Sinus tracts
Acetic acid	0.5%−5% acetic acid solution	Infected wound caused by *Pseudomonas aeruginosa*	Noninfected wounds or infection of other origins
Sodium hypochlorite	Sodium hypochlorite 0.25% solution or Dakin's solution. Bactericidal effect on Gram-negative bacteria	Infection control in pressure ulcers Dissolving necrotic tissue	Harmful to healthy tissue Nonnecrotic wounds
Povidone-iodine	Topical antiseptic solution effective on Gram-positive and Gram-negative bacteria. Causes dry skin and stain on surrounding tissues	Surgical hand scrub Infected wounds	Prolonged application Large wounds Wounds in patient with thyroid disorders
Chlorhexidin	2% chlorhexidin solution effective on Gram-positive and Gram-negative bacteria May cause hypersensitivity, including anaphylaxis, generalized urticaria, bronchospasm, cough, dyspnea, wheezing, and malaise	Surgical hand scrub Infected wounds	Wounds in face or head due to damage to the eye and middle ear
Silver nano colloidal solution	Odorless and colorless silver nano colloidal solution with no irritation and effective on a wide range of pathogenic viruses, bacteria, and fungi	Surgical hand scrub Infected wounds	Can be applied on all type of wounds and intact skin

WOUND TREATMENT

Wound healing is a complex biological process, which influences multiple tissue types. Tissue regeneration aims to repair damaged tissue and replace it with new ones that are physiologically and functionally similar to the original tissue [48].

Tissue regeneration, as one of the major areas of regenerative medicine, has been developed to make up for donor tissue shortages, tissue replacement rejections, and the delayed or stopped inflammatory phase. Wound tissue regeneration strategies have been focused on providing moisturized environments, accelerating the inflammatory response, quality granulation tissue formation, and infection control. Modern methods provide an appropriate space to facilitate cellular activities (i.e., migration and proliferation) and evoke the soluble mediators to accelerate tissue regeneration [1−4].

Precise wound staging and infection status determination are necessary for accurate prescription. On the other hand, it is crucial for wound care professionals to consider the cost-effectiveness and availability of the treatment methods.

In this chapter, the modern wound treatment approaches have been discussed briefly as follows:

Modern wound dressings, skin grafts, stem cells therapy, platelet-rich plasma, ozone therapy, hyperbaric oxygen therapy, negative pressure wound therapy, low-level laser therapy, and artificial skin. Fig. 5.2 represents a classification of various wound healing techniques.

These methods have been developed to facilitate wound healing process through different mechanisms, e.g., providing adequate wound moisture and key factors for granulation tissue formation (growth factors, cytokines, etc.), tissue oxygenation, and antibacterial activity.

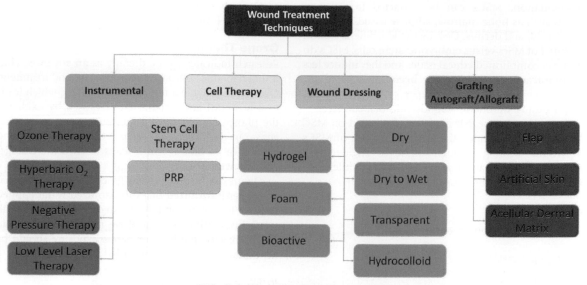

FIG. 5.2 Wound treatment techniques.

Functional requirements for these methods are as follows:

1. Biocompatibility
2. Providing moisturized environment
3. Pain relief
4. Exudate management
5. Odor management
6. Prevention and control of infection
7. Antiscar effect

Skin Graft

Skin graft is a surgical procedure consisting of removing and transferring an area of healthy skin of various thickness and size for covering skin loss of other parts of the body due to nonhealing complex wounds such as chronic ulcers and full-thickness burns [49,50].

Early reports of skin grafting as one of the standard treatments for wound care date back to more than 2000 years ago carried out by Indians [51] (Fig. 5.3).

Skin grafts are classified into two categories based on thickness of the explant:

1. split-thickness skin graft contains only a section of the dermis
2. full-thickness skin graft contains the whole dermis [52].

Indications

- Sufficient blood supply to the wound bed

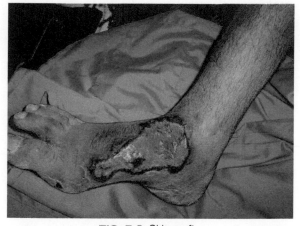

FIG. 5.3 Skin graft.

Contraindications

- Necrotic wound
- Poor blood supply
- Exposed bone or tendon
- Vessels or nerve without soft tissue coverage
- Implanted biomaterials without soft tissue support
- Stressed locations (e.g., joints, heel, neck)
- Local infection [53].

Stem Cell Therapy

Mesenchymal stem cells (MSCs) are adult stem cells with the ability of self-renewal and multipotential differentiation. MSCs can be extracted from many tissues such as bone marrow, adipose tissue, umbilical cord blood, and dermis. Despite the less differentiation potential of MScs versus embryonic stem cells, MSCs do not meet complicated ethical issues and they induce less immunoreactions. MSCs have been investigated for skin regeneration in various types of wound such as burn wounds, traumatic wounds, and diabetic ulcers.

Considerable research has been conducted on MSC therapy, which revealed the synergistic effect of MSCs on wound healing through enhanced angiogenesis, reepithelialization, and tissue granulation, while these mechanisms have yet to be elucidated [54,55].

Indications
- Nonhealing chronic wound

Contraindications
- Necrotic wound
- Chronic infection
- Vasculitis
- Terminal stages of disease
- Advanced metabolic disorder
- Cancer and metastasis [56]

Platelet-Rich Plasma
Platelet-rich plasma (PRP) is blood plasma enriched with concentrate of autologous platelet, derived from whole blood. PRP represents a natural source of cytokines and growth factors, such as PDGF, TGF-β, VEGF, and bFGF, which encourage tissue regeneration [57].

Currently, due to easy processing, efficiency, and predictable manner, PRP has been widely used to accelerate the healing process for many applications, such as wound healing, plastic surgery, dentistry, and orthopedics. PRP acts as a tissue sealant with the ability of local release of proteins and growth factors, which trigger cellular migration, differentiation, and proliferation. In addition, PRP regulates the cytokines and facilitates the angiogenesis and reepithelialization in chronic wounds. Some researchers have been reported the antibacterial effect of PRP [58,59].

Indications
- Small to medium size wounds

Contraindications
- Necrotic wound
- Thrombocytopenia
- Platelet dysfunction syndrome

- Hemodynamic instability
- Anemia [60]

Ozone Therapy
Research indicates ozone therapy as an advanced clinical therapeutic approach for chronic wound treatment. Ozone can provide a mild oxidative stress, which leads to a powerful antibacterial effect caused by oxidizing the phospholipids and lipoproteins inside the pathogens. On the other hand, ozone raises the H−O and N−O level in blood, which leads to elicit the endogenous growth factors.

Ozone can be delivered by gaseous exposure (mixed by oxygen), ozonized oil, and ozonized water applied directly to the wound or indirect exposure through rectal insufflation. It should be noted that, to avoid ozone toxicity, the level of ozone exposure should be kept under a therapeutic limit [61,62].

Indications
- All infected wounds
- Diabetic foot ulcers

Contraindications
- Face and neck wounds
- Long-term use due to toxic inhalation of ozone

Hyperbaric Oxygen Therapy
Hyperbaric oxygen therapy (HBOT) is an advanced therapeutic technique, in which patients are placed inside a chamber, and then they breathe high-pressure pure oxygen for a short time. In recent decades, HBOT is commonly used for treatment of different types of wound including diabetic foot ulcers, chronic wounds, and posttraumatic wounds. However, high cost, side effects, and inaccessible equipment caused that the usage of topical oxygen therapy (TOT) for wound healing becomes more popular than HBOT. TOT is a technique of delivering pure oxygen to the damaged tissues at an atmospheric pressure slightly above 1 atm. Oxygen influences the signal transduction pathways of multiple growth factors, including those involved in propagating angiogenesis [63−65].

Indications
- Nonhealing chronic wound
- Osteomyelitis
- Necrotic wound

Contraindications
- Pneumothorax
- COPD

- Acute viral infection
- Congenital spherocytosis
- Uncontrolled acute seizures disorder
- Upper respiratory tract infection [66,67]

Negative Pressure Wound Therapy

Negative-pressure wound therapy (NPWT) is a noninvasive clinical therapeutic approach for wound healing. NPWT applies an adjustable subatmospheric pressure on the wound site through a sealed dressing connected to a vacuum pump. NPWT accelerates the healing process and wound contraction in acute or chronic wounds by reducing interstitial edema, increasing angiogenesis, draining wound exudate, and encouraging blood circulation [68,69].

Indications

- Chronic wound
- Burn wound
- Fistula

Contraindications

- Osteomyelitis
- Necrotic wound
- Malignant wound

Low-Level Laser Therapy

Low-level laser therapy (LLLT) also known as low-intensity laser therapy (LILT) is a noninvasive therapeutic technique by applying the red and near infrared light on the wound. LLLT stimulate the cells and activates wound healing pathways by increasing granulation tissue formation, fibroblast proliferation, collagen synthesis, neovascularization, and early epithelialization. LLLT can be an effective treatment for nonhealing diabetic ulcers and hypertrophic scars [70–72].

Indications

- Surgical wound
- Chronic wound

Contraindications

- Vasodilation
- Wound over the eye
- Malignant lesions
- Wound over the thyroid gland
- Patient with epilepsy [73]

WOUND DRESSINGS

In recent years, wound dressings have been widely used to facilitate wound healing. They typically replace the damaged tissues, and provide a moisturized environment for appropriate cell migration thereby resulting in minimal scar tissue formation. These dressings range from antibacterial woven pads to growth factor in situ forming gels. Fig. 5.4 compares the wound healing process in a wound covered by a hydrogel dressing with a wound left without any treatment.

In the last decades, the use of biocompatible polymers from different sources has been investigated for medical, biomedical, and pharmaceutical applications. Many biocompatible polymers have been developed for wound healing applications, which have addressed promising results in tissue regeneration. The multifunctional behavior and flexible nature of biopolymers make them an appropriate treatment for a wide variety of wound types in different condition, e.g. wounds with excess exudate or dry wounds, which need absorbing and hydrating dressings, respectively [74].

An ideal dressing is defined according to the wound conditions. For example, for a very dry wound, it should donate moisture to the wound bed, while for a highly exuding wound it should absorb excess exudate and there is no miracle dressing which could heal all wounds, therefore top wound care companies offer specialized dressings for different stages of wound.

Bioactive Dressing

Bioactive wound dressings are either made of substances which release bioactive compounds or alternatively natural biomaterials having endogenous activity are used in their constructions. These biomaterials may include chitin, chitosan, hydrocolloids, alginate or derivatives of natural biopolymers.

Dry Dressing

Traditionally, dry dressings are known as woven or nonwoven gauze pads or common bandages. Dry dressings are easy to use, highly permeable, nonocclusive and inexpensive, and provide relatively trauma protection, bacterial barrier, and pain relief. Usually, dry dressings adhere to the wound surface; therefore, to avoid granulation tissue damaging or bleeding, it is necessary to moisturize the dressing with water or normal saline before changing it.

Indications

- Surgical incisions and abrasions of any size, and depth.

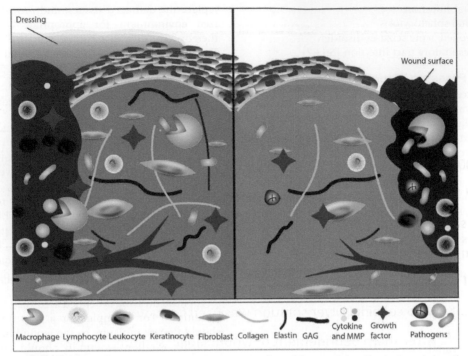

Dressing

Wound surface

Macrophage Lymphocyte Leukocyte Keratinocyte Fibroblast Collagen Elastin GAG Cytokine and MMP Growth factor Pathogens

FIG. 5.4 Effect of dressing on the quality of wound healing. After applying the hydrogel, keratinocyte migration, growth factors regulation, and vascularization will improve due to providing moist environment. In addition, the dressing acts as a physiochemical barrier against microorganisms.

Contraindications

- Necrotic wound
- Granular wound bed [3,22,75]

Wet-to-Dry Dressing

Wet-to-dry dressings are semipermeable, pliable, woven or nonwoven films, or moist gauze dressing with adhesive backing. They are permeable to vapor while impermeable to bacteria. The primary moist layer poorly absorbs wound exudate, while the layer donates water molecules to the wound surface, which results in necrotic tissue and wound debris removal by changing the dressing. To avoid maceration, a secondary dry dressing should be applied on the primary dressing.

Indications

- Mechanical debridement
- Necrotic wound

Contraindications

- Infected wound
- Wound with moderate to heavy exudate
- Fragile skin [3,22,75]

Transparent Dressing

Transparent dressings are impermeable, nondegradable, and adhesive dressing that enable the wound observation without changing the dressing.

Indications

- Clean debrided nonbleeding wound
- Laparoscopic incision
- Superficial wound
- Graft donor site with minimal drainage

Contraindications

- Infected wounds
- Wounds with moderate to heavy exudate [3,22,75]

Hydrocolloid Dressing

Hydrocolloid dressings are generally composed of hydrophilic colloidal particles (e.g., gelatin, cellulose) embedded within an adhesive film or foam. The wafer-shape structure of hydrocolloid dressing enables the interaction between the particles and wound exudates that results in the swelling of the dressing and forming a soft barrier against urine, stool, and pathogens. Hydrocolloid dressings are impermeable to gas, vapor, water, and bacteria, and their transparent appearance enables the wound observation and checking the wound exudate. Most of the hydrocolloid dressings may leave residue in the wound bed.

Indications
- Moderate exuding wound
- Pressure ulcers
- Wound under compression wraps

Contraindications
- Bleeding wound
- Wounds with heavy exudate
- Some of the hydrocolloid dressings are not suitable for infected wound
- Undermining, tunneling, or sinus tract [3,22,75]

Hydrogel Dressing
The main component of hydrogel dressings is water entrapped within a cross-linked polymeric network; therefore, they poorly absorb fluid, while they donate a large amount of moisture to dry or necrotic wounds. These dressings are available in various forms, such as film, gel, or impregnated mesh-type dressing, which are permeable to gas, vapor, and water. They provide a soft barrier against shear force, act as a shock-absorbing pad, and reduce the patient's pain.

The periwound areas must be watched for excess moist and maceration. Most of the hydrogel dressings are nonadhesive and need a protective secondary dressing.

Indications
- Wound with minimal or moderate drainage
- Pressure ulcer
- Partial/full-thickness wound
- Graft donor site
- Vascular ulcer
- Skin tear
- Dermabrasion
- Radiation burn

Contraindications
- Infected wound
- Wound with heavy exudate [3,22,75]

Foam Dressing
Foam dressings are commonly composed of polyurethane, which may be coated by a very thin contact layer. They are absorbent and are permeable to gas, vapor, and water. The hydrophilic porous structure of the foam dressings enables the exudate absorption several times greater than their initial weight. They provide a flexible and soft bed for wounds over bony prominences or friction areas. In an appropriate timely manner, they can be applied on infected wounds.

Indications
- Wound over bony prominences or friction areas
- Partial/full thickness wound
- Granular wound bed
- Skin tear
- Graft donor site
- Wound under compression wraps
- Surgical incision
- Infected wound
- Wound with moderate to heavy exudate

Contraindications
- Dry wound
- Eschar wound
- Burn wound [3,22,75]

Dressing Materials
This atlas provides an overview on the physiochemical properties and biological effects of several important biopolymers (e.g., sodium alginate, calcium alginate, and chitosan) as wound dressings.

Alginates
The most widely used polysaccharide in wound healing is alginate. Alginate is a general term for a family of polysaccharides produced by seaweed, brown algae, and bacteria.

Alginate is a heteropolysaccharide made from two randomly arranged uronic acid and sugar molecules (i.e., G blocks and M blocks).

Generally, alginates with more G blocks have stiffer chains in comparison with alginates that have more M-blocks, which suggest a more flexible structure with more swelling capacity. The two uronic acids can bind to metal ions, such as sodium and calcium, which are widely used in the alginate dressings formulation [76].

Calcium Alginate. Calcium alginate is the insoluble form of alginate with high swelling capacity. It can be woven to produce pliable patches or ribbons for filling cavity or tunneling wounds.

Calcium alginate has the potential to absorb 15—20 times more than its initial weight, and its nonadhesive surface makes it possible to be easily removed from the wound site [74].

Sodium Alginate. The extent of swelling is directly related to the calcium/sodium ratio. The sodium alginate donates water molecules out of its initial network, due to the greater tendency of sodium ions to bond with G blocks, which leads to a more dense structure. Therefore, sodium ions releasing from alginate can be suggested as an effective water delivery pump for moisturizing the wound environment, particularly in necrotic tissues or dry wounds.

Chitosan
Chitosan is the generic family of polycationic derivatives of poly-N-acetyl-D-glucosamine (chitin), which is found in the external layer of crustacean body, and in the fungi and bacteria cell walls.

Chitosan is naturally a weak base, and insoluble at neutral or alkaline pH. It is a biodegradable, nontoxic, nonimmunogenic, and biocompatible biopolymer, and has received a great deal of attention in cosmetic, food, pharmaceutical, and biomedical industries.

Chitosan accelerates wound healing through polymorphonuclear cells and fibroblast activation, cytokine production, giant cell migration and stimulation of type IV collagen synthesis, wound moisturizing, and antimicrobial nature due to positive charge.

The adhesive nature of chitosan, together with the antimicrobial feature, and oxygen permeability, make it a very useful material for wound dressing. On the other hand, chitosan facilitates the granulation tissue formation in open wounds and organizes the collagen fibers rearrangement in the remodeling phase. Different derivatives of chitin and chitosan have been prepared to fulfill the different needs for a variety of wound healing applications in multiple forms, including hydrogels, fibers, membranes, powder, and sponges [74,76].

Dressing Selection
After wound assessment, appropriate dressings should be selected based on wound size, depth, exudate, stage, infection status, the patient age and general condition. There is no predetermined principle for selecting the appropriate dressing, while some important factors should be considered before the dressing selection, such as price, availability, medical team experience, and preference of the patient and medical team.

DEBRIDEMENT
Debridement is the removal of devitalized, infected, or damaged tissue from the wound surface to accelerate wound healing. As mentioned before, necrotic tissue provides an ideal environment for pathogen replication and impairs wound healing; hence, debridement is an important part of wound care management. The aim of debridement is the removal of devitalized and sever-contaminated tissues with no damage to the living surrounding tissues, for example, nerves, vessels, tendons, bones, and muscles.

Debridement accelerates wound healing by enabling the wound bed assessment and infection control. The main components of necrotic tissue are avascular tissue, fibrinous exudate, and bacteria or other pathogens.

It should be noted that for ischemic wounds, debridement is harmful to the wound tissue and it is contraindicated. Therefore, it is crucial to evaluate the blood perfusion, particularly in patients suspected to peripheral arterial disease [22,75].

There are several methods for debridement, which are classified into invasive and minimally invasive methods (Fig. 5.5).

Indications for Debridement
- Necrotic tissue
- Contamination or infection
- As an adjunct with other treatment methods [3,22,75,77]

Surgical Debridement
Surgical debridement is the fastest, highly selective, and most aggressive debridement method, which is applied by sharp instruments such as scalpels, scissors, laser, and hydrosurgical water knife. The success of surgical debridement is highly depended on the level of skill and knowledge of the physician or nurse, and it should be done in wound care centers or operating rooms. Bleeding, infection, and general complications after anesthesia are possible side effects of surgical debridement. Fig. 5.6 shows the removal of necrotic tissue via surgical debridement.

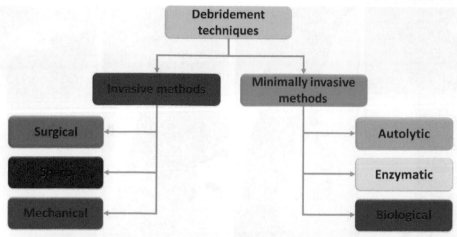

FIG. 5.5 Debridement techniques.

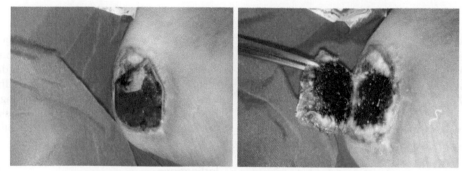

FIG. 5.6 Surgical debridement for a pressure ulcer in an operating room.

Indications

- Osteomyelitis
- Infectious arthritis
- Ascending cellulitis
- Extensive necrotic tissue
- Wound with urgent need for debridement, for example, necrotic tissue near vital organs

Contraindications

- Malignant wound
- Patient with coagulation disorders
- Ischemia
- Immunocompromised patient [3,22,75,77]

Sharp Debridement

Sharp debridement refers to the selective and fast removal of necrotic tissues, foreign materials, and debris from the wound bed by using forceps, scissor, or scalpel. Sharp debridement is the fastest and the second most aggressive debridement technique after surgical debridement. It must be performed by wound-expert professionals who are highly skilled in using sharp instruments. Fig. 5.7 shows the sharp debridement process, which is performed by a home care therapist.

Indications

- Progressive cellulitis or sepsis
- Necrotic tissue (eschar or slough)
- Callus tissue

Contraindications

- Noninfected ischemic ulcer
- Wound with insufficient blood supply

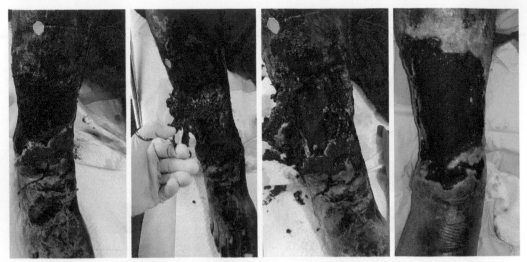

FIG. 5.7 Sharp debridement for a chronic traumatic ulcer.

- Wound with unclear interface between viable and nonviable tissue
- Patients who are on anticoagulant therapy
- Immunosuppressed or thrombocytopenic patient [3,22,75,77]

Mechanical Debridement

Mechanical debridement, as the oldest debridement method, describes the use of mechanical force to remove devitalized tissue, foreign bodies, and debris from the wound bed. It suggests a nonselective technique due to the removal of nonspecific areas of devitalized tissue.

There are several techniques for applying the certain amount of force for mechanical debridement with minimized trauma, including wet-to-dry dressings, scrubbing, and whirlpool.

The mechanical force of water jet provides the required force for debridement in wound irrigation, pulsatile lavage, and whirlpool techniques.

Wet-to-Dry Dressing

Applying wet-to-dry dressings is a common debridement method, in which a moist saline gauze dressing is placed on the wound surface and is left to dry. The removal of the dried gauze results in the removal of devitalized tissue and debris from the wound bed.

Despite the advantages of the wet-to-dry technique such as low cost, it may hurt the surrounding viable tissue during the removal of the dressing, and cause extreme pain, bleeding, wound bed desiccation, and periwound maceration; therefore, the other methods of debridement are generally preferred.

Indications

- Infected wound

Contraindications

- Noninfected wound
- Patient with low pain tolerance
- Wound with granulation tissue [3,22,75]

Hydrotherapy

Hydrotherapy (i.e., whirlpool) debridement is indicated for patients with large wounds who need aggressive cleaning or softening of the necrotic tissue. It is contraindicated in granulating wounds because it can macerate and injure the wound bed [3,22,75].

Autolytic Debridement

Autolytic debridement is a highly selective technique in which moisture-retentive dressings are used to soften the necrotic tissue by moist donation from dressing and body fluid and digest it by endogenous enzymes, neutrophils, and phagocytes.

Autolytic debridement as a minimally invasive method is safe and cost-effective. It causes minimal pain, which makes it suitable for patients with low pain tolerance, but it is a time-consuming process. Autolytic debridement can be performed by patient or caregivers with low expertise but the wound should be watched carefully for maceration. Figs. 5.8 and 5.9 show autolytic debridement process without and with macerated wound edges, respectively.

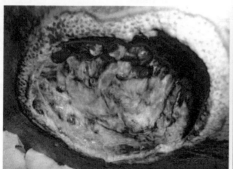 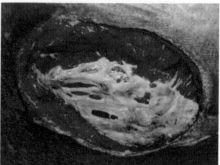

FIG. 5.8 Autolytic debridement without wound edge maceration.

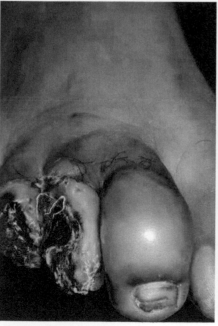 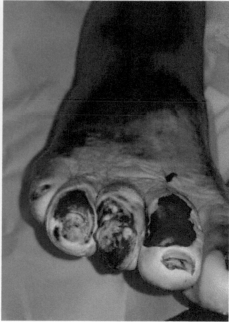

FIG. 5.9 Autolytic debridement with macerated wound edges, which can impair wound healing and make the skin more vulnerable to infection.

Indications

- Noninfected wound with necrotic tissue
- Patient who cannot tolerate other debridement methods
- Home-care or long-term care debridement settings

Contraindications

- Wound with urgent need for debridement
- Infected wound
- Extensive or deep cavity wound
- Wound that require sharp or surgical debridement
- Severe neutropenia
- Immunocompromised patients [3,22,75,77]

Enzymatic and Chemical Debridement

Enzymatic debridement refers to a selective method in which three main exogenous enzymes: proteolytics, fibrinolytics and collagenases, are used for devitalized tissue removal. Unlike the sharp and surgical debridement, it causes less pain but takes more time. Chemical debridement refers to removing necrotic tissue by chemical agents such as sodium hypochlorite and hydrogen proxide. Some references use enzymatic and chemical debridement, interchangeably because in both of them the necrotic tissue is digested through chemical reactions, but they are different in the nature of the digesting agent. Enzymatic debridement is limited due to high cost and low availability.

It should be noted that prophylactic infection is commonly reported during enzymatic debridement; therefore, it must be performed by health-expert professional under supervision of physician for rapid diagnosis of infection.

Indications

- Patient who cannot tolerate sharp debridement
- Home-care or long-term care debridement settings

Contraindications

- Wound with exposed deep tissues such as bone and tendon
- Wound requiring rapid debridement
- Facial wounds
- Calluses (enzymes are unable to debride calluses) [3,22,75,77]

Biological Debridement

Biological debridement, also known as larval or maggot therapy, is performing selective debridement by using maggots as live medical devices. The sterilized maggots are placed on the wound surface within a net pouch, and fixed by an absorbent dressing. Wound debridement is performed by maggot through two mechanisms:

1. Secreting proteolytic enzymes, which soften and degrade the necrotic tissue with no damage to healthy tissue
2. Ingesting the necrotic tissue and bacteria

Indications

- Infected wound
- Wound with granulation tissue

Contraindications

- Patient allergic to adhesives, fly larvae, eggs, and soybeans
- Patient with coagulation disorder
- Deep tunneling wound
- Active pyoderma gangrenosum in the absence of proper treatment
- Wound likely to communicate to the central nervous system, large blood vessels, body cavities, or vital organs
- In necrotizing or rapidly advancing infection (necrotizing fasciitis, gaseous gangrene)
- Sepsis [3,22,75,77]

SCAR TISSUE MANAGEMENT

Patients, health care professionals, and researchers are all concerned about unpleasant scar appearance; hence, selecting an appropriate strategy for wound treatment is crucial to minimize the scar tissue formation.

Scar Tissue

Scar tissue formation, as a normal part of wound healing, initiates in proliferation phase, continues after remodeling phase, and may cause unpleasant appearance and/or disruption in normal functioning. It occurs at the termination of wound healing process and lasts from 4 weeks to years. It is a physiologic response to an injury deep in the dermis.

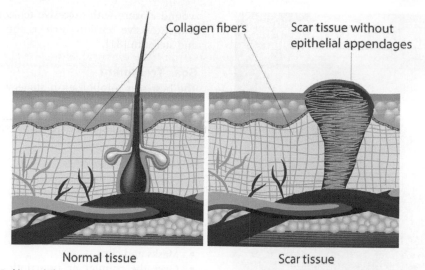

Collagen fibers

Scar tissue without epithelial appendages

Normal tissue

Scar tissue

FIG. 5.10 Normal tissue versus scarred tissue. Collagen fibers are formed in tiled pattern in normal tissue, while formed parallelized in scar tissue, which is results in more stiffness in scar tissue. Furthermore, the skin appendages, for example, hair follicles, sebaceous glands, and sweat glands, are disappeared in scar tissue.

Typically, a mature scar is composed of arranged collagen fibers parallel to the skin surface orientation, but in normal skin, collagen fibers form a basket weave-like network. Due to lack of rete pegs,[1] the basement membrane at the epidermis—dermis interface, which is covering the scar tissue, is flatter than the one of normal skin. Furthermore, typical skin appendages such as hair follicles and sweat glands do not develop on scar tissue [3,78]. Fig. 5.10 shows the difference between normal tissue and scar tissue schematically.

After scar maturation, the decreased population of fibroblasts along with the lack of skin appendages leads to form the dermis layer with a small number of cells. The ECM in normal skin contains more elastin fibers comparing to the scar tissue; therefore, scar tissue behaves less elastic. Finally, contractures formation caused by activity of fibroblasts and myofibroblasts can be painful and will restrict movement especially when the scar is located over a joint [78,79]. Figs. 5.11 and 5.12 show normal and hypertrophic scar tissues, respectively. Clinical characteristics of different types of scar tissues, namely normal, hypertrophic, and keloid, are summarized in Table 5.2.

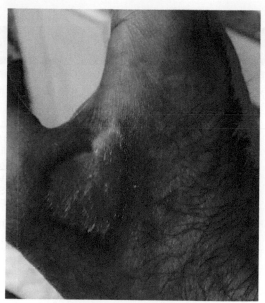

FIG. 5.11 Normal scar.

Both hypertrophic scarring and keloids are extended beyond the borders of initial wound and are more vascularized, with thicker epidermal layers comparing to the normal scar tissue. Hypertrophic scar is more probable to occur after wound infection,

---

[1]Rete pegs are the epithelial extensions in the underlying connective tissue at the interface of epidermis and dermis.

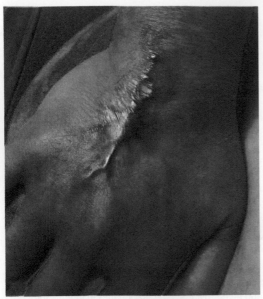

FIG. 5.12 Hypertrophic scar.

wound closure with excessive tension, and locations with excessive tension such as the shoulders, neck, and sternum [81].

Scar Treatment

The best scar minimization strategy suggests primary prevention, but in some cases, scarring is unavoidable and requires secondary intervention. The main treatment approaches are as follows:

Noninvasive Approach

- Compression therapy and occlusive dressing (pressure garments with or without gel sheeting)
- Static and dynamic splints
- Silicone gel or films
- Acrylic casts
- Masks and clips
- Over the counter or prescription of a variety of ointments, oils, lotions, and creams
- Hydrotherapy
- Massage therapy

TABLE 5.2
Clinical Characteristics of Different Types of Scar Tissue [78–80]

Scar Tissue	Raising	Color	Characteristics	Onset	ECM
Normal	Lower than the surrounding skin	White to pink	Soft, shiny	Within weeks, tends to regress with time	Parallel collagen fibers
Hypertrophic	Slightly higher than the surrounding skin	White to pink or red	Firm, itchy, painful, follows the wound borders	Within weeks or months, tends to regress with time	Wavy bundles of collagen. More collagen fibers and ground substance and less elastin fibers than normal scar
Keloid	Very raised	Deep red to purple	Firm, extended beyond the wound borders	Within years, tends to progress with time	Disorganized bundles of irregular collagen fibers. More ground substance and less elastin fibers than hypertrophic scar

**Acute Wound Treatment Algorithm
(Fig. 5.13)**

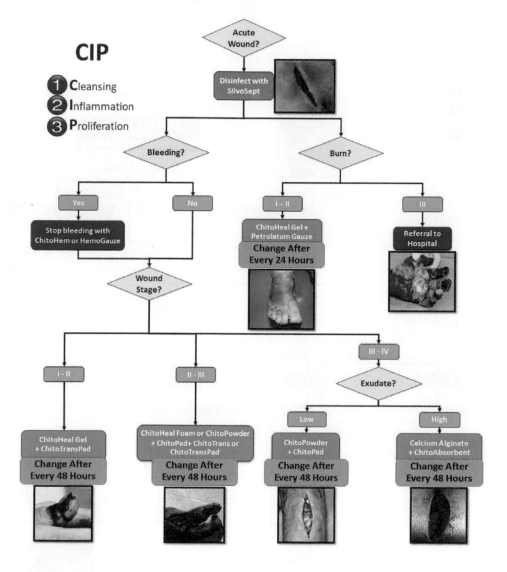

❦ Always disinfect the wound with SilvoSept before applying the dressing.

❦ After wound closure, continue treatment with applying ChitoScar every 24 hours.

FIG. 5.13 Acute wound treatment algorithm (CIP).

Chronic Wound Treatment Algorithm
(Fig. 5.14)

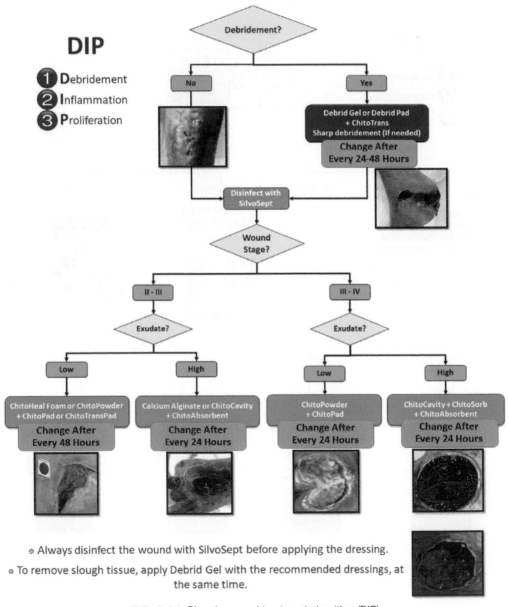

FIG. 5.14 Chronic wound treatment algorithm (DIP).

Invasive Treatments

- Surgical excision and resuturing
- Intralesional corticosteroid injection and other pharmacological options including fluorouracil, interferon gamma, bleomycin, doxorubicin, verapamil, retinoic acid, tamoxifen, and tacrolimus
- Radiotherapy

- Laser therapy
- Cryosurgery

In some cases, the scar tissue is left without treatment for a year, to observe the progression and make a decision [80,82].

a. Acute Wound Treatment Algorithm
b. Chronic Wound Treatment Algorithm

CHAPTER 6

Wound Classification

There is no universal classification for wounds, and several classification methods are presented for categorizing the wounds. Three of the most practical classifications are shown in Fig. 6.1. The most important parameters for wound classification are the nature of wound cause, duration (whether acute or chronic), and the depth of injury to the skin and underlying tissues [83,84].

ACUTE WOUNDS

An acute wound refers to a breakdown of the integrity of the soft tissue, which occurs suddenly and heals by a predictable timely manner. Acute wounds are usually healed by primary intention.

The acute wound might be simple or complex, depending on its location, size, involved anatomic structures, and bioburden. Traumatic wounds and surgical wounds are examples of acute wounds [85].

CHRONIC WOUNDS

Wound healing is a complex process and involves many biological pathways. Tissue regeneration can be negatively affected by multiple factors such as infection, concurrent disease (e.g., diabetes, vascular disease, and cancer), malnutrition, in the presence of which, wound fails to heal and develops to chronic ulcer.

When an acute wound fails to heal in a predictable timely manner (4–6 weeks), a chronic wound occurs, in which healing process could be delayed, stopped or worsen over time. Chronic wounds require secondary intention to activate the healing process. Pressure ulcers, diabetic foot ulcers, and venous ulcers are the major types of chronic wounds.

Systemic reasons such as chronic debilitation, malnourishment, diabetes, and sepsis may cause chronic wounds, but in all cases, acute wound healing cascade

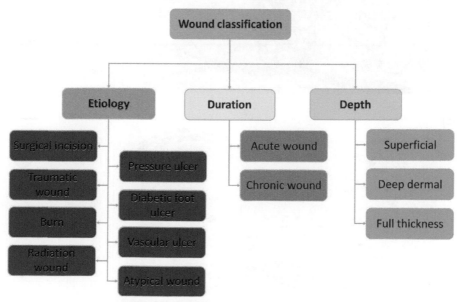

FIG. 6.1 Different classifications of wound.

Atlas of Wound Healing. https://doi.org/10.1016/B978-0-323-67968-8.00006-9

is affected by a local factor. Chronic wounds are characterized by high levels of proteolytic enzymes and cytokines, which inhibit the granulation tissue formation and epithelialization. Remaining in this phase provides an ideal environment for bacterial colonization, and healing process may be interrupted by infection [85,86]. Table 6.1 and Fig. 6.2 indicate the differences between acute and chronic wounds.

TABLE 6.1
Characteristics of Acute and Chronic Wounds [85–87]

Acute Wounds	Chronic Wounds
Treatment duration less than a month	Unhealed within 6 weeks of formation
No underlying pathology	Underlying pathology
Normal inflammatory stage	Prolonged inflammatory stage
Usually heals without complication	Variety of complication
Acute wound fluid supports cell proliferation	Chronic wound fluid does not support cell proliferation
Presence of TGF-β	Degradation of TGF-β
Increased concentration of PDGF, FGF and VEGF	Decreased concentration or lack of PDGF, FGF and VEGF

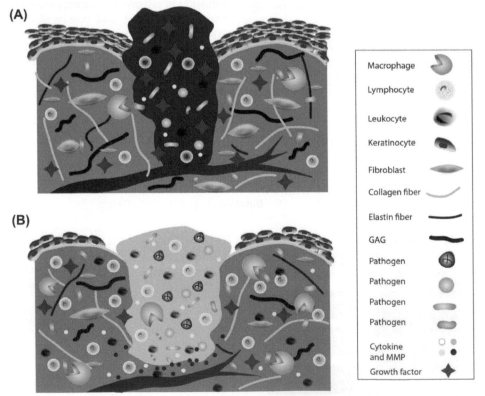

FIG. 6.2 The differences between acute and chronic wounds: the significant increase in population of keratinocytes and fibroblasts as well as more growth factors and less pathogens in acute wound **(A)** versus chronic wound **(B)**.

CHAPTER 7

Pressure Ulcers

According to the National Pressure Ulcer Advisory Panel (NPUAP): "A pressure ulcer is localized damage to the skin and/or underlying soft tissue usually over a bony prominence. The ulcer can present as intact skin or an open ulcer and may be painful. The ulcer occurs because of intense and/or prolonged pressure or pressure in combination with shear. The tolerance of soft tissue for pressure and shear may also be affected by microclimate, nutrition, perfusion, comorbidities and condition of the soft tissue." The NPUAP classifies the pressure ulcer according to the tissue loss [88]. Fig. 7.1 presents a schematic staging of pressure ulcer.

STAGE I

Stage I pressure ulcer is characterized by nonblanchable erythema of the intact skin usually over a bony prominence. It may be painful, soft, firm, or warmer than surrounding tissue. It may appear differently in dark skin people (Fig. 7.2).

STAGE II

Stage II pressure ulcer is characterized by partial-thickness skin loss with pink or red exposed dermis. The wound bed is moist, viable, and without slough tissue. In some cases, Stage II pressure ulcer might appear as an intact or raptured blister (Fig. 7.3).

STAGE III

Stage III pressure ulcer refers to full-thickness tissue loss, in which adipose tissue may be visible. This stage is characterized by granulation tissue and epibole (rolled wound edges) formation, while in some cases slough or eschar tissue may be appeared. The wound depth varies by wound site, and undermining and tunneling may occur. Underlying tissues such as muscle, tendon, and bone are not exposed (Fig. 7.4).

STAGE IV

Stage IV pressure ulcer is characterized by full-thickness skin and tissue loss, with exposed muscle, tendon, ligament, cartilage or bone, and slough or eschar tissue formation. Epibole (rolled edges), undermining, and/or tunneling may occur (Fig. 7.5).

UNSTAGEABLE PRESSURE ULCER (DEPTH UNKNOWN)

Unstageable pressure ulcer refers to obscured full-thickness skin and tissue loss in which the extent of tissue damage within the ulcer cannot be confirmed because it is obscured by slough or eschar. When slough or eschar tissue is removed, a Stage III or IV pressure ulcer will be revealed. In presence of stable eschar (i.e., dry and adherent necrotic tissue, without erythema or fluctuance) on the heel or ischemic limb, debridement is contraindicated (Fig. 7.6).

SUSPECTED DEEP TISSUE INJURY (DEPTH UNKNOWN)

Suspected deep tissue injury is characterized by a localized area of maroon or purple discoloration with blood-filled blister, while skin remained intact. In some cases, pain and temperature change precede skin color changes. Discoloration may appear differently in dark skin people. This injury can be a result of intense or prolonged pressure or shear forces at the bone—muscle interface. It may develop to apparent wound, or may disappear without tissue loss (Fig. 7.7).

Wound Care Management and Early Treatment for Pressure Ulcer

1. Inspect wound once a day.
2. Use moisturizer for dry skin.
3. Avoid massage over bony prominences.
4. Use proper position and turning techniques.
5. Use barriers to reduce friction injuries.
6. Schedule bathing; avoid hot water and cleansing agents.
7. Rehabilitation program.
8. Apply antiseptic solutions and provide appropriate wound dressing, according to the degree of ulcer.

Atlas of Wound Healing. https://doi.org/10.1016/B978-0-323-67968-8.00007-0

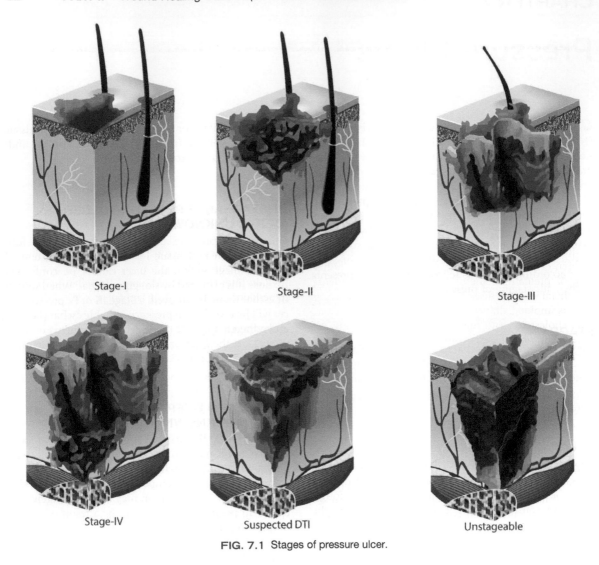

Stage-I   Stage-II   Stage-III

Stage-IV   Suspected DTI   Unstageable

FIG. 7.1 Stages of pressure ulcer.

FIG. 7.2 Stage I pressure ulcer.

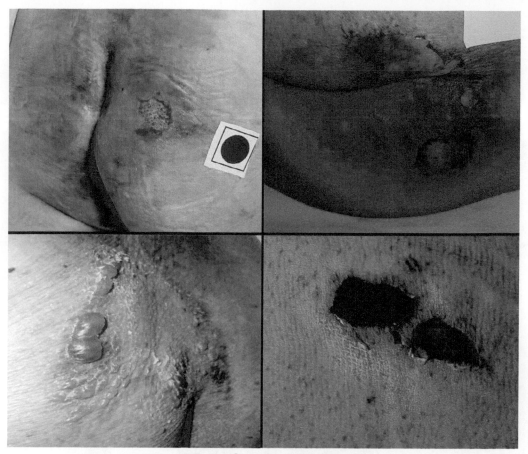

FIG. 7.3 Stage II pressure ulcer.

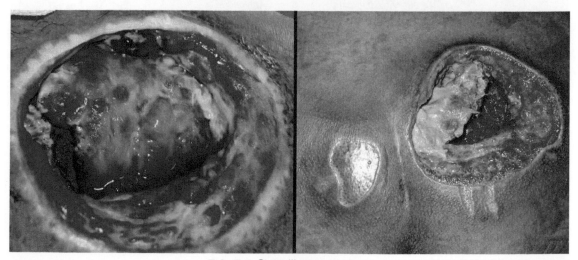

FIG. 7.4 Stage III pressure ulcer.

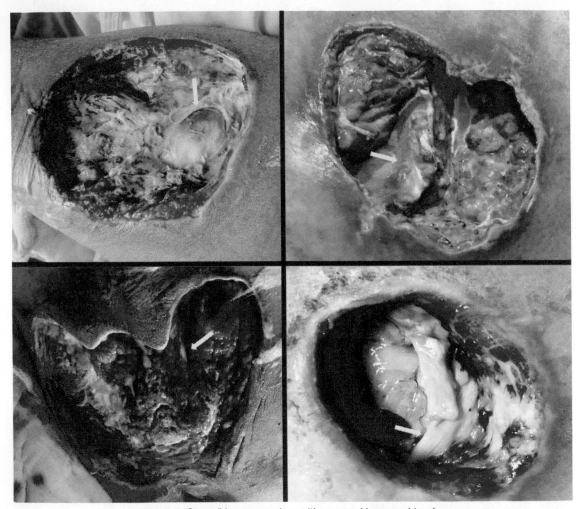

FIG. 7.5 Stage IV pressure ulcer with exposed bone and tendon.

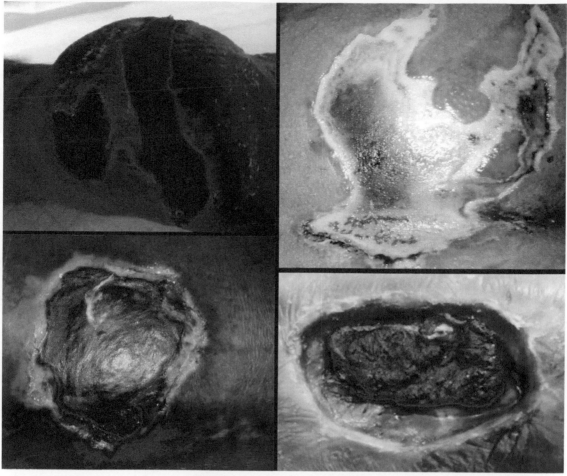

FIG. 7.6 Unstageable pressure ulcer.

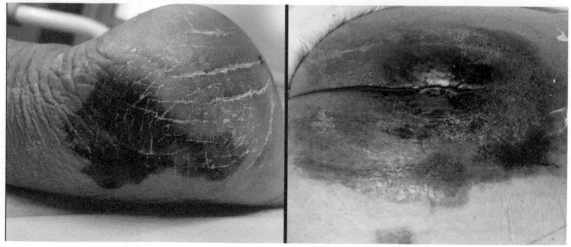

FIG. 7.7 Suspected deep tissue injury (DTI).

Case Reports

Figs. 7.8 to 7.47 show the treatment process for different stages of pressure ulcer.

Stage-I Pressure Ulcer

Year: 2018

Age and Sex: 58, F

Wound site: Buttock

Duration of treatment: 5 days

Cause of wound: Hospitalization after CVA.

Treatment: Nano colloidal silver solution was used for wound disinfection. Chitosan gel was applied to make a barrier to prevent wound progress.

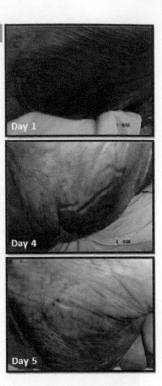

FIG. 7.8 Pressure ulcer.

Stage-II Pressure Ulcer

Year: 2018

Age and Sex: 49, M

Wound site: Right shoulder

Duration of treatment: 8 days

Cause of wound: Hospitalization due to cancer to receive chemotherapy.

Treatment: Nano colloidal silver solution was used for wound disinfection. Chitosan gel was used for tissue regeneration.

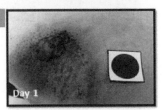
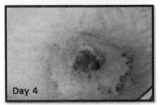
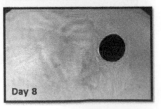

FIG. 7.9 Pressure ulcer.

Stage-II Pressure Ulcer

Year: 2018

Age and Sex: 25, M

Wound site: Buttock

Duration of treatment: 10 days

Cause of wound: Immobilization after car accident.

Treatment: Nano colloidal silver solution was used for wound disinfection. Chitosan gel was used for tissue regeneration.

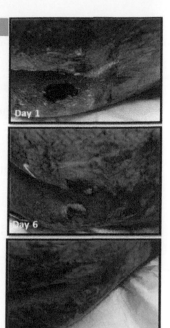

FIG. 7.10 Pressure ulcer.

Stage-II Pressure Ulcer

Year: 2017

Age and Sex: 27, M

Wound site: Sacral region

Duration of treatment: 11 days

Cause of wound: Hospitalization after intoxication.

Treatment: Nano colloidal silver solution was used for wound disinfection. Chitosan gel was applied for tissue regeneration.

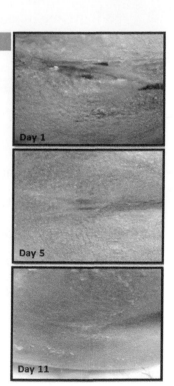

FIG. 7.11 Pressure ulcer.

Stage-II Pressure Ulcer

Year: 2017

Age and Sex: 85, M

Wound site: Sacral region

Duration of treatment: 30 days

Cause of wound: Hospitalization after CVA.

Treatment: Nano colloidal silver solution was used for wound disinfection. Chitosan gel was applied for tissue regeneration.

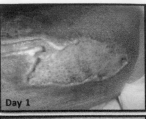
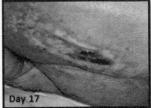
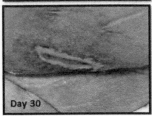

FIG. 7.12 Pressure ulcer.

Stage-II Pressure Ulcer

Year: 2015

Age and Sex: 77, M

Wound site: Left trochanter

Duration of treatment: 10 days

Cause of wound: Hospitalization after CVA.

Treatment: Nano colloidal silver solution was used for wound disinfection. Chitosan gel was applied for tissue regeneration.

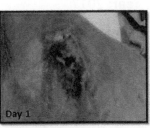
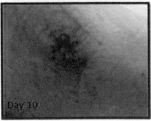

FIG. 7.13 Pressure ulcer.

Stage-II Pressure Ulcer

Year: 2014

Age and Sex: 58, M

Wound site: Buttock

Duration of treatment: 12 days

Cause of wound: Immobilization after an open heart surgery.

Treatment: Nano colloidal silver solution was used for wound disinfection. Chitosan gel was applied for tissue regeneration.

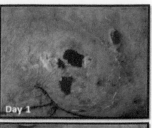
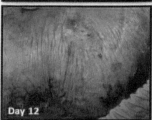

FIG. 7.14 Pressure ulcer.

Stage-II Pressure Ulcer

Year: 2014

Age and Sex: 82, M

Wound site: Right trochanter

Duration of treatment: 16 days

Cause of wound: Hospitalization after CVA.

Treatment: Nano colloidal silver solution was used for wound disinfection. Chitosan gel was applied for tissue regeneration.

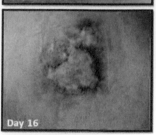
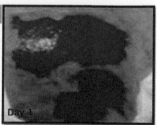

FIG. 7.15 Pressure ulcer.

Stage-II Pressure Ulcer

Year: 2014

Age and Sex: 73, M

Wound site: Right trochanter

Duration of treatment: 15 days

Cause of wound: Hospitalization after CVA.

Treatment: Nano colloidal silver solution was used for wound disinfection. Chitosan gel was applied for tissue regeneration.

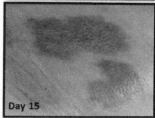

FIG. 7.16 Pressure ulcer.

Stage-II Pressure Ulcer

Year: 2014

Age and Sex: 76, F

Wound site: Right trochanter

Duration of treatment: 26 days

Cause of wound: Hospitalization after CVA.

Treatment: Nano colloidal silver solution was used for wound disinfection. Chitosan gel was applied for tissue regeneration.

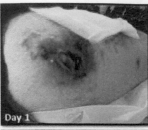
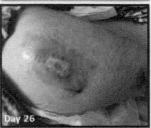

FIG. 7.17 Pressure ulcer.

Stage-II Pressure Ulcer

Year: 2006

Age and Sex: 11, M

Wound site: Right buttock

Duration of treatment: 10 days

Cause of wound: Immobilization after car accident.

Treatment: Nano colloidal silver solution was used for wound disinfection. Chitosan gel was applied for tissue regeneration.

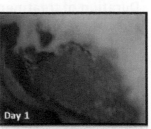
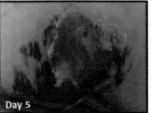
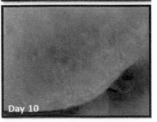

FIG. 7.18 Pressure ulcer.

Stage-II Pressure Ulcer

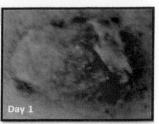

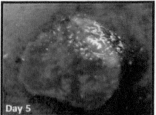

Year: 2006

Age and Sex: 76, M

Wound site: Buttock

Duration of treatment: 9 days

Cause of wound: Hospitalization after CVA.

Treatment: Nano colloidal silver solution was used for wound disinfection. Chitosan gel was applied for tissue regeneration.

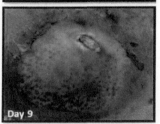

FIG. 7.19 Pressure ulcer.

Stage-III Pressure Ulcer

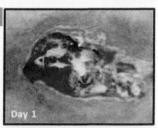

Year: 2018

Age and Sex: 58, M

Wound site: Sacral region

Duration of treatment: 75 days

Cause of wound: Immobilization after car accident.

Treatment: Nano colloidal silver solution was used for wound disinfection. Sodium alginate and chitosan powder were used for autolytic debridement and tissue regeneration, respectively.

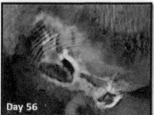

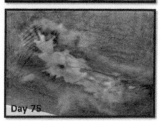

FIG. 7.20 Pressure ulcer.

Stage-III Pressure Ulcer

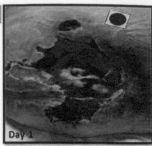

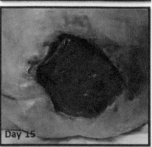

Year: 2018

Age and Sex: 40, M

Wound site: Sacral region

Duration of treatment: 15 days

Cause of wound: Immobilization due to spinal cord injury.

Treatment: Nano colloidal silver solution was used for wound disinfection. Sodium alginate and chitosan powder were used for autolytic debridement and tissue regeneration, respectively.

FIG. 7.21 Pressure ulcer.

Stage-III Pressure Ulcer

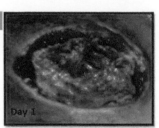

Year: 2017

Age and Sex: 27, F

Wound site: Sacral region

Duration of treatment: 55 days

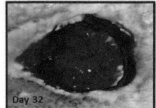

Cause of wound: Hospitalization after renal failure.

Treatment: Nano colloidal silver solution was used for wound disinfection. Sodium alginate and chitosan powder were used for autolytic debridement and tissue regeneration, respectively.

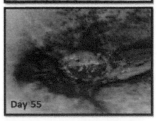

FIG. 7.22 Pressure ulcer.

Stage-III Pressure Ulcer

Year: 2017

Age and Sex: 73, M

Wound site: Right trochanter

Duration of treatment: 45 days

Cause of wound: Brace therapy pressure.

Treatment: Nano colloidal silver solution was used for wound disinfection. Sodium alginate and chitosan (gel and powder) were used for autolytic debridement and tissue regeneration, respectively.

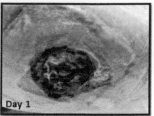
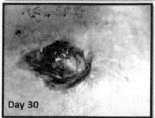
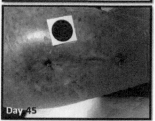

FIG. 7.23 Pressure ulcer.

Stage-III Pressure Ulcer

Year: 2016

Age and Sex: 35, M

Wound site: Groin region

Duration of treatment: 75 days

Cause of wound: Immobilization after car accident.

Treatment: Nano colloidal silver solution was used for wound disinfection. Sodium alginate and chitosan powder were used for autolytic debridement and tissue regeneration, respectively.

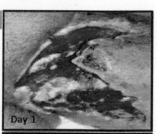
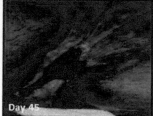
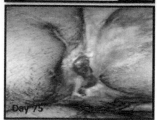

FIG. 7.24 Pressure ulcer.

Stage-III Pressure Ulcer

Year: 2015

Age and Sex: 70, M

Wound site: Right trochanter

Duration of treatment: 30 days

Cause of wound: Hospitalization after CVA.

Treatment: Nano colloidal silver solution was used for wound disinfection. Sodium alginate and chitosan (gel and powder) were used for autolytic debridement and tissue regeneration, respectively.

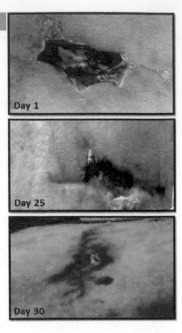

FIG. 7.25 Pressure ulcer.

Stage-III Pressure Ulcer

Year: 2014

Age and Sex: 92, M

Wound site: Sacral region

Duration of treatment: 80 days

Cause of wound: Hospitalization after CVA.

Treatment: Nano colloidal silver solution was used for wound disinfection. Sodium alginate and chitosan (gel and powder) were used for autolytic debridement and tissue regeneration, respectively.

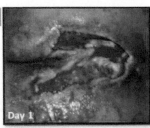
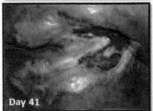
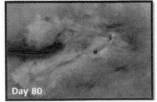

FIG. 7.26 Pressure ulcer.

Stage-III Pressure Ulcer

Year: 2014

Age and Sex: 77, F

Wound site: Sacral region

Duration of treatment: 75 days

Cause of wound: Hospitalization after CVA.

Treatment: Nano colloidal silver solution was used for wound disinfection. Sodium alginate and chitosan (gel and powder) were used for autolytic debridement and tissue regeneration, respectively.

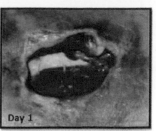
Day 1

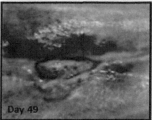
Day 49

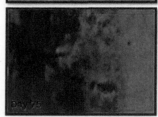
Day 75

FIG. 7.27 Pressure ulcer.

Stage-III Pressure Ulcer

Year: 2014

Age and Sex: 76, M

Wound site: Medial side of right knee

Duration of treatment: 21 days

Cause of wound: Hospitalization after CVA.

Treatment: Nano colloidal silver solution was used for wound disinfection. Sodium alginate and chitosan (gel and powder) were used for autolytic debridement and tissue regeneration, respectively.

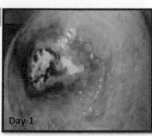
Day 1

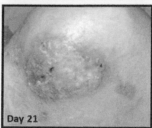
Day 21

FIG. 7.28 Pressure ulcer.

Stage-III Pressure Ulcer

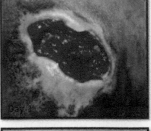
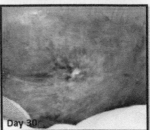

Year: 2005

Age and Sex: 71, M

Wound site: Sacral region

Duration of treatment: 30 days

Cause of wound: Hospitalization after CVA.

Treatment: Nano colloidal silver solution was used for wound disinfection. Chitosan gel and powder were used for tissue regeneration.

FIG. 7.29 Pressure ulcer.

Stage-IV Pressure Ulcer

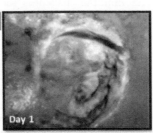
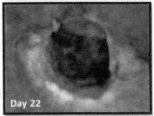

Year: 2005

Age and Sex: 47, F

Wound site: Sacral region

Duration of treatment: 90 days

Cause of wound: Immobilization after car accident.

Treatment: Nano colloidal silver solution was used for wound disinfection. Sodium alginate and chitosan (gel and powder) were used for autolytic debridement and tissue regeneration, respectively.

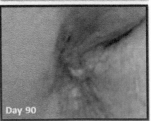

FIG. 7.30 Pressure ulcer.

Stage-IV Pressure Ulcer

Year: 2005

Age and Sex: 30, F

Wound site: Sacral region

Duration of treatment: 60 days

Cause of wound: Immobilization due to MS.

Treatment: Nano colloidal silver solution was used for wound disinfection. Patient was treated by traditional dressing for one month and underwent a surgical debridement without any improvement. Sodium alginate and chitosan (powder, foam and gel) were applied for autolytic debridement and tissue regeneration, respectively.

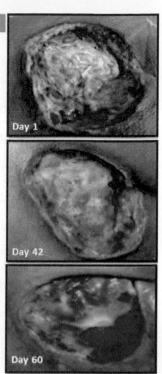

FIG. 7.31 Pressure ulcer.

Stage-IV Pressure Ulcer

Year: 2005

Age and Sex: 30, F

Wound site: Right trochanter

Duration of treatment: 60 days

Cause of wound: Immobilization due to MS.

Treatment: Nano colloidal silver solution was used for wound disinfection. Patient was treated by traditional dressing for one month and underwent a surgical debridement without any improvement. Sodium alginate and chitosan (powder, foam and gel) were applied for autolytic debridement and tissue regeneration, respectively.

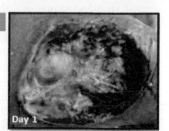
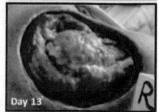
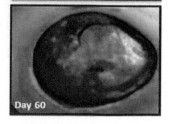

FIG. 7.32 Pressure ulcer.

Stage-IV Pressure Ulcer

Year: 2005

Age and Sex: 30, F

Wound site: Left trochanter

Duration of treatment: 60 days

Cause of wound: Immobilization due to MS.

Treatment: Nano colloidal silver solution was used for wound disinfection. Patient was treated by traditional dressing for one month and underwent a surgical debridement without any improvement. Sodium alginate and chitosan (powder, foam and gel) were applied for autolytic debridement and tissue regeneration, respectively.

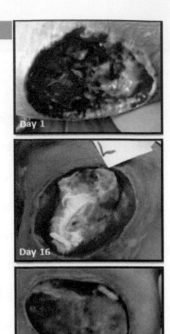

FIG. 7.33 Pressure ulcer.

DTI Pressure Ulcer

Year: 2016

Age and Sex: 68, M

Wound site: Sacral region

Duration of treatment: 40 days

Cause of wound: Hospitalization after an open heart surgery.

Treatment: Nano colloidal silver solution was used for wound disinfection. Chitosan foam and gel were applied to treat the ulcer while keeping an eye on suspected DTI. Treatment was successful with no DTI developing.

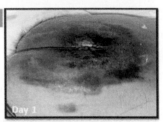

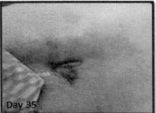

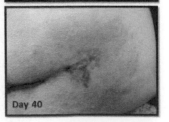

FIG. 7.34 Pressure ulcer.

Unstageable Pressure Ulcer

Year: 2017

Age and Sex: 47, F

Wound site: Right leg

Duration of treatment: 65 days

Cause of wound: Immobilized after knee arthroplasty.

Treatment: Nano colloidal silver solution was used for wound disinfection. Sodium alginate was used for autolytic debridement along with sharp debridement. After removal of necrotic tissue, the ulcer was diagnosed as stage-III pressure ulcer. Treatment was continued with chitosan powder and gel.

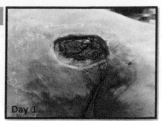
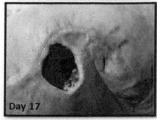
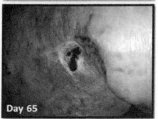

FIG. 7.35 Pressure ulcer.

Unstageable Pressure Ulcer

Year: 2017

Age and Sex: 79, M

Wound site: Sacral region

Duration of treatment: 63 days

Cause of wound: Hospitalization after CVA.

Treatment: Nano colloidal silver solution was used for wound disinfection. Sodium alginate was used for autolytic debridement along with sharp debridement. After removal of necrotic tissue, the ulcer was diagnosed as stage-IV pressure ulcer. Treatment was continued with sodium alginate, chitosan (powder, foam and gel) for autolytic debridement of residual slough and tissue regeneration, respectively. Patient expired.

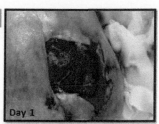
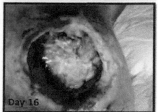
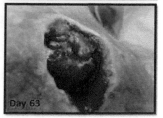

FIG. 7.36 Pressure ulcer.

Unstageable Pressure Ulcer

Year: 2017

Age and Sex: 87, F

Wound site: Sacral region

Duration of treatment: 31 days

Cause of wound: Hospitalization after CVA.

Treatment: Nano colloidal silver solution was used for wound disinfection. Sodium alginate was used for autolytic debridement along with sharp debridement. After removal of necrotic tissue, the ulcer was diagnosed as stage-III pressure ulcer. Treatment was continued with sodium alginate, chitosan (powder, and gel) for autolytic debridement of residual slough and tissue regeneration, respectively.

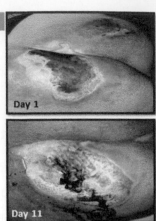
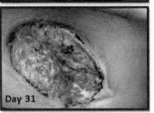
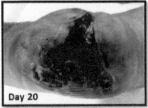

FIG. 7.37 Pressure ulcer.

Unstageable Pressure Ulcer

Year: 2017

Age and Sex: 28, M

Wound site: Right heel

Duration of treatment: 65 days

Cause of wound: Immobilization due to spinal cord injury.

Treatment: Nano colloidal silver solution was used for wound disinfection. Sodium alginate was used for autolytic debridement along with sharp debridement. After removal of necrotic tissue, the ulcer was diagnosed as stage-II pressure ulcer. Treatment was continued with chitosan foam and gel.

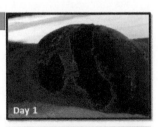
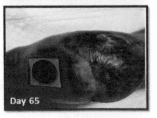

FIG. 7.38 Pressure ulcer.

Unstageable Pressure Ulcer

Year: 2017

Age and Sex: 32, F

Wound site: Sacral region

Duration of treatment: 76 days

Cause of wound: Immobilization due to spinal cord injury.

Treatment: Nano colloidal silver solution was used for wound disinfection. Sodium alginate was used for autolytic debridement along with sharp debridement. After removal of necrotic tissue, the ulcer was diagnosed as stage-III pressure ulcer. Treatment was continued with chitosan powder and gel.

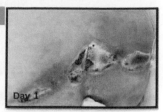
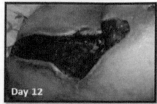
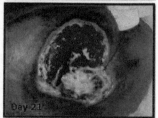

FIG. 7.39 Pressure ulcer.

Unstageable Pressure Ulcer

Year: 2017

Age and Sex: 86, F

Wound site: Sacral region

Duration of treatment: 65 days

Cause of wound: Hospitalization after CVA.

Treatment: Nano colloidal silver solution was used for wound disinfection. Sodium alginate was used for autolytic debridement along with sharp debridement. After removal of necrotic tissue, the ulcer was diagnosed as stage-III pressure ulcer. Treatment was continued with calcium alginate.

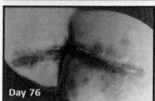
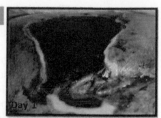
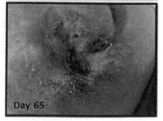

FIG. 7.40 Pressure ulcer.

Unstageable Pressure Ulcer

Year: 2016

Age and Sex: 81, M

Wound site: Sacral region

Duration of treatment: 90 days

Cause of wound: Hospitalization after CVA.

Treatment: Nano colloidal silver solution was used for wound disinfection. Sodium alginate was used for autolytic debridement along with sharp debridement. After removal of necrotic tissue, the ulcer was diagnosed as stage-III pressure ulcer. Treatment was continued with sodium alginate, chitosan (powder, and gel) for autolytic debridement of residual slough and tissue regeneration, respectively.

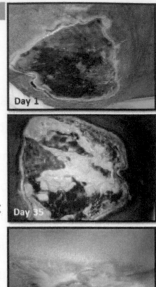

FIG. 7.41　Pressure ulcer.

Unstageable Pressure Ulcer

Year: 2016

Age and Sex: 85, M

Wound site: Heel of right foot

Duration of treatment: 56 days

Cause of wound: Hospitalization after CVA.

Treatment: Nano colloidal silver solution was used for wound disinfection. After surgical debridement sodium alginate was used for autolytic debridement. After removal of necrotic tissue, the ulcer was diagnosed as stage-II pressure ulcer. Treatment was continued with calcium alginate and chitosan gel for tissue regeneration.

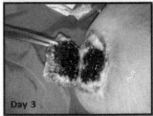

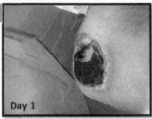

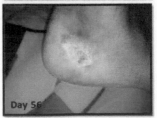

FIG. 7.42　Pressure ulcer.

Unstageable Pressure Ulcer

Year: 2016

Age and Sex: 81, M

Wound site: Sacral region

Duration of treatment: 65 days

Cause of wound: Hospitalization after CVA.

Treatment: Nano colloidal silver solution was used for wound disinfection. Sodium alginate was used for autolytic debridement along with sharp debridement. After removal of necrotic tissue, the ulcer was diagnosed as stage-II pressure ulcer. Treatment was continued with calcium alginate.

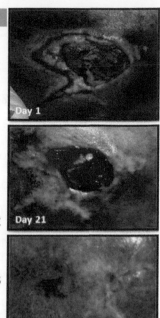

FIG. 7.43 Pressure ulcer.

Unstageable Pressure Ulcer

Year: 2016

Age and Sex: 28, M

Wound site: Sacral region

Duration of treatment: 60 days

Cause of wound: Immobilization due to spinal cord injury.

Treatment: Nano colloidal silver solution was used for wound disinfection. Sodium alginate was used for autolytic debridement along with sharp debridement. After removal of necrotic tissue, the ulcer was diagnosed as stage-III pressure ulcer. Treatment was continued with sodium alginate, chitosan (powder, and gel) for autolytic debridement of residual slough and tissue regeneration, respectively.

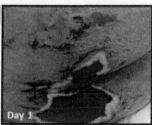

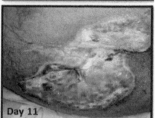

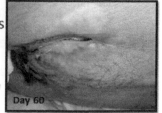

FIG. 7.44 Pressure ulcer.

Unstageable Pressure Ulcer

Year: 2006

Age and Sex: 64, F

Wound site: Sacral region

Duration of treatment: 25 days

Cause of wound: Hospitalization after heart attack.

Treatment: Nano colloidal silver solution was used for wound disinfection. Sodium alginate was used for autolytic debridement along with sharp debridement. After removal of necrotic tissue, the ulcer was diagnosed as stage-III pressure ulcer. Treatment was continued with sodium alginate, chitosan (powder, and gel) for autolytic debridement of residual slough and tissue regeneration, respectively. Patient expired.

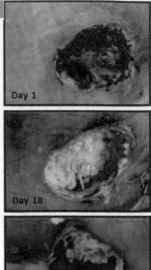
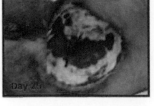

FIG. 7.45 Pressure ulcer.

Unstageable Pressure Ulcer

Year: 2006

Age and Sex: 33, F

Wound site: Left thigh

Duration of treatment: 45 days

Cause of wound: Immobilized due to congenital hemiplegia.

Treatment: Nano colloidal silver solution was used for wound disinfection. Sodium alginate was used for autolytic debridement along with sharp debridement. After removal of necrotic tissue, the ulcer was diagnosed as stage-III pressure ulcer. Treatment was continued with chitosan powder and gel.

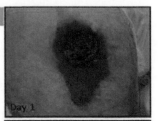
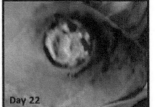
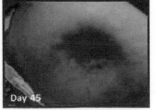

FIG. 7.46 Pressure ulcer.

Unstageable Pressure Ulcer

Year: 2005

Age and Sex: 82, M

Wound site: Sacral region

Duration of treatment: 30 days

Cause of wound: Hospitalization after CVA.

Treatment: Nano colloidal silver solution was used for wound disinfection. Sodium alginate was used for autolytic debridement along with sharp debridement. After removal of necrotic tissue, the ulcer was diagnosed as stage-IV pressure ulcer. Treatment was continued with sodium alginate, chitosan (powder, and foam) for autolytic debridement of residual slough and tissue regeneration, respectively. Patient expired.

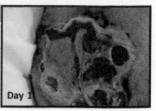
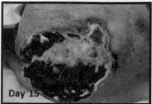
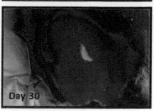

FIG. 7.47 Pressure ulcer.

CHAPTER 8

Diabetic Foot Ulcers

Diabetes is a metabolic disorder characterized by hyperglycemic conditions that is associated with functional abnormalities of insulin secretion and/or defective insulin activity [89].

The global burden of diabetes has been rising rapidly, and it is estimated that currently more than 425 million people suffer from diabetes all over the world, increasing to 628 million by 2045 [90].

The chronic hyperglycemia can cause long-term damages and subsequently failure of various organ systems [91]. Diabetic foot ulcer (DFU) is one of the most common complications of diabetes, which is a result of peripheral neuropathy (PN) and peripheral vascular disease (PVD) of the lower limb [92].

It has been reported that 19%—34% of patients with diabetes will probably experience DFU in their life, and the International Diabetes Federation estimated that foot ulcers affect 9.1 to 26.1 million people with diabetes annually all over the world. On the other hand, 1% of diabetic patients undergo an amputation worldwide every year [93]. Fig. 8.1 represents foot amputation following DFU.

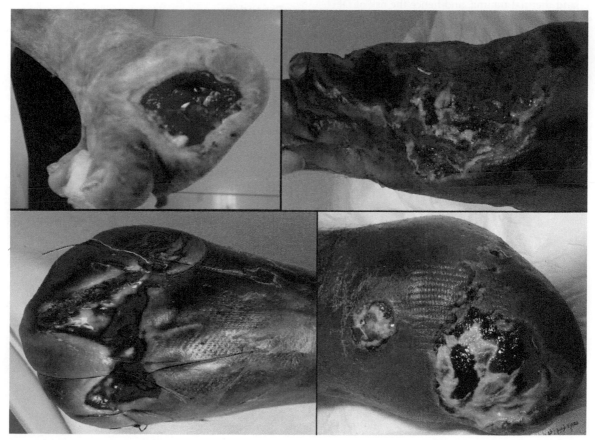

FIG. 8.1 DFU leads to amputation in 1% of patients every year.

Atlas of Wound Healing. https://doi.org/10.1016/B978-0-323-67968-8.00008-2

PATHOPHYSIOLOGY OF DFU

DFU is a result of multiple factors including peripheral neuropathy, peripheral vascular disease, that is, ischemia, and infection [94].

Diabetic Peripheral Neuropathy

Diabetic peripheral neuropathy (DPN) is one of the main causes of DFU, and it is estimated that around half of the diabetic patients experience peripheral neuropathy [95].

The increase in blood glucose level gradually damages blood vessels and nerves, which leads to poor circulation and neuropathy [96]. Foot deformity, limited joint mobility, unusual foot pressure, and subsequently callus development over pressure points occur as the result of neuropathy. There are three different types of neuropathy as follows:

- **Sensory Neuropathy**, the most common type of neuropathy, leads to loss of protective sensation (i.e., pain), which increases susceptibility to physical and thermal trauma, and hence the risk of DFU.
- **Motor Neuropathy** is characterized by atrophy, muscle imbalance, and structural foot deformity such as hammertoe, hallux rigidus and limited joint mobility.
- **Autonomic Neuropathy** is characterized by decreased sweating, fissures, dry and shiny skin, and foot is vulnerable to small trauma [97,98].

The combination of sensory and motor neuropathy causes a nonpainful chronic ulcer of the sole of the foot due to bony projections that is called Malum perforans pedis [99] (Fig. 8.2).

Moreover, neuroarthropathy leads to Charcot foot, which is a chronic painless progressive degenerative arthropathy resulting from disturbance in sensory innervation of the affected joints. Charcot foot can be characterized by deformity, redness, swelling, increased temperature, and ulceration [94,98] (Fig. 8.3).

DFU ASSESSMENT

Several methods can be performed to identify sensory neuropathy, such as Semmes-Weinstein test and vibration perception threshold. On the other hand, ankle–brachial index and ultrasound Doppler have been widely used to investigate the peripheral tissue perfusion.

Semmes-Weinstein Test

This test aims to determine the degree of sensory neuropathy.

Procedure

1. Use a 10 g monofilament to assess the test and touch the patient's arm and hand to show what it feels like.
2. Ask the patient to close their eyes.
3. Touch the testing point by monofilament tip and press it to make a C shape, as shown in Fig. 8.4.
4. Ask the patient to say yes when they feel touched by monofilament on their feet.

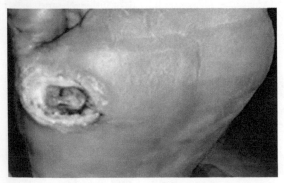

FIG. 8.2 Malum perforans pedis.

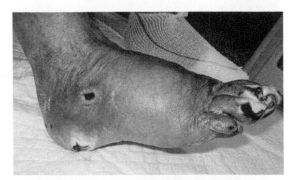

FIG. 8.3 DFU with deformed foot, i.e., Charcot.

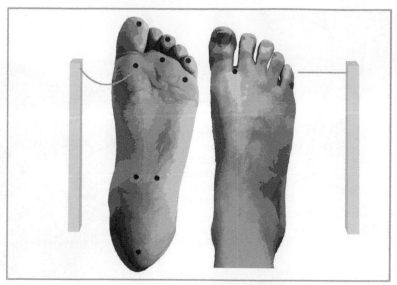

FIG. 8.4 Assessing the sensory neuropathy using monofilament.

If the patient does not feel the monofilament at any site, it means that they lost the protective sensation at that point.

Ankle–Brachial Index

The ankle–brachial index (ABI) also known as the toe–brachial index (TBI) refers to a fast, reliable, noninvasive technique for assessing the peripheral tissue perfusion and peripheral arterial disease (PAD). The ABI measurement is the most widely used technique for determining the healing potential in diabetic foot patients.

The ABI ratio is obtained by dividing the higher of the ankle pressures for each leg by the higher of the right and left arm's brachial systolic pressures. Normal ABI is in the range of 0.9−1.1 [100].

Doppler Ultrasound Probing

Doppler ultrasound, as a noninvasive technique, has been widely used for assessing arterial patency, when peripheral pulses are not easily palpable to predict the healing potential in DFU. Doppler probing evaluates the blood flow inside the vessel by Doppler Effect of ultrasound waves. A transmitting probe sends an input signal, which is reflected with a different intensity. In vessel with nonpalpable pulsation, the output Doppler signal descends and detects the poor blood perfusion inside the vessel [3,22].

DFU Grading

The Wagner−Meggit system is the most widely used grading system for DFU, which is composed of six grades since 25 years ago. It focuses on the depth of ulcer, presence of gangrene, and level of tissue necrosis (Fig. 8.11). Wagner Grades 0 to 5 are as follows:

Grade 0—Intact Skin, no open lesions or cellulitis (Fig. 8.5)

Grade 1—Superficial ulcer of skin or subcutaneous tissue (Fig. 8.6)

Grade 2—Ulcers extend into tendon, bone, or capsule (Fig. 8.7)

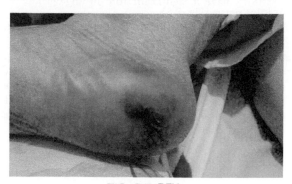

FIG. 8.5 DFU.

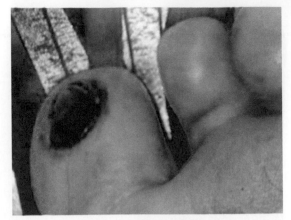

FIG. 8.6 Grade 1 DFU.

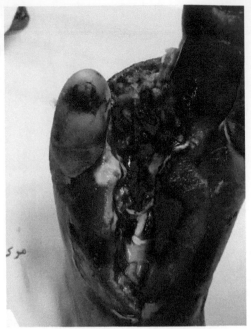

FIG. 8.8 Grade 3 DFU.

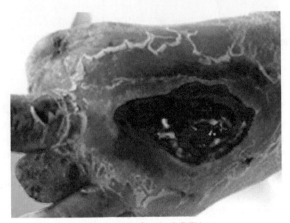

FIG. 8.7 Grade 2 DFU.

Grade 3—Deep ulcer with osteomyelitis, abscess, and/or joint sepsis (Fig. 8.8)
Grade 4—Partial foot gangrene, that is, local gangrene forefoot or heel (Fig. 8.9)
Grade 5—Whole foot gangrene (Fig. 8.10)
    Furthermore, DFU can be classified clinically based on the degree of neuropathy and vascular damage, as neuropathic, neuroischemic, and ischemic diabetic ulcers. The clinical characteristics of the three major types of DFU are presented in Table 8.1.

WOUND CARE MANAGEMENT AND EARLY TREATMENT FOR DFU

1. Check etiology and risk factors
2. Assess the degree of neuropathy (Semmes-Weinstein test)
3. Noninvasive vascular assessment (ABI)
4. For diabetic neuropathy, off-loading is vital for treating and preventing the ulcer.
5. In case of soft tissue infection, start oral antibiotics treatment under medical supervision.
6. In case of osteomyelitis, hospitalization is suggested and IV antibiotics treatment.
7. Autolytic debridement is suggested for ischemic or neuroischemic ulcers, while mechanical debridement is highly recommended for neuropathic ulcer.
8. Autolytic debridement is recommended in presence of slough tissue.
9. Apply antiseptic solutions, and provide appropriate wound dressing according to ulcer degree.

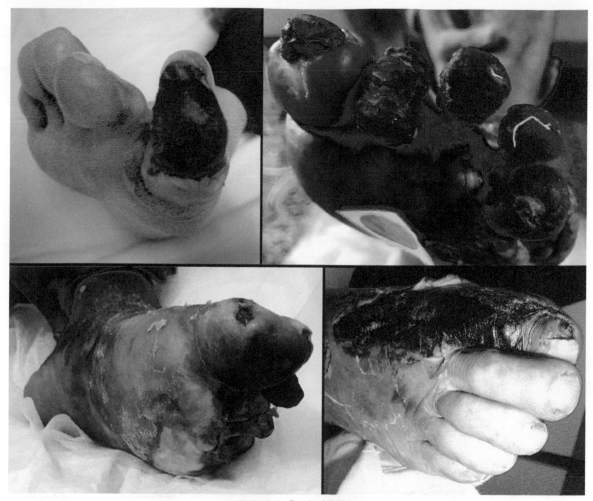

FIG. 8.9 Grade 4 DFU.

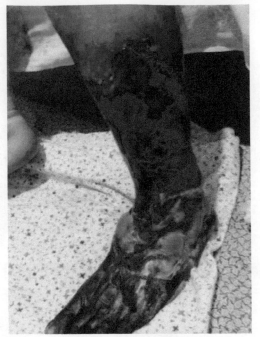

FIG. 8.10 Grade 5 DFU.

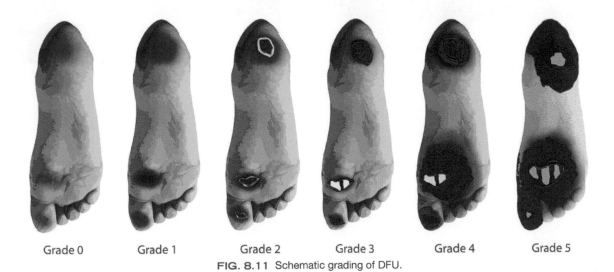

| Grade 0 | Grade 1 | Grade 2 | Grade 3 | Grade 4 | Grade 5 |

FIG. 8.11 Schematic grading of DFU.

TABLE 8.1
Clinical Characteristics of Three Major Types of DFU (Neuropathic, Ischemic, and Neuroischemic) [94]

Ulcer Characteristics	Ischemic	Neuroischemic	Neuropathic
Common location	Borders	Sole, toes, heel, borders	Sole, toes, heel
Wound tissue type	Necrotic	Necrotic and callus	Callus
Pain	Severe	Dull pain	Mild
Sensation	Present	Absent or present	Absent
Bone deformity	Absent	Present	Present
Arterial pulses	Weak or absent	Weak or absent	Present
Temperature	Cool	Cool	Warm
Sweating	Present	Absent or present	Absent
Appearance	Hairless, necrosis, thin, and shiny skin	Yellow callus	Dry, fissure, and callus

CASE REPORTS

Figs. 8.12—8.44 show the treatment process for DFU.

Diabetic Foot Ulcer

Year: 2018

Age and Sex: 54, F

Wound site: Left big toe

Duration of treatment: 47 days

Cause of wound: Ischemia.

Treatment: Nano colloidal silver solution was used for wound disinfection. Sodium alginate and chitosan gel were used for autolytic debridement and tissue regeneration, respectively.

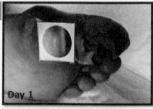
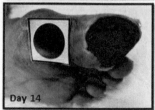
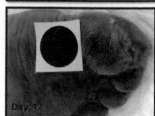

FIG. 8.12 DFU.

Diabetic Foot Ulcer

Year: 2018

Age and Sex: 60, Male

Wound site: Left foot

Duration of treatment: 42 days

Cause of wound: Neuropathic DFU due to contact with a hot object.

Treatment: Nano colloidal silver solution was used for wound disinfection. Sodium alginate was used for autolytic debridement. After removal of necrotic tissue, treatment was continued with chitosan gel and calcium alginate for tissue regeneration.

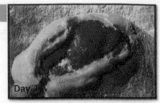
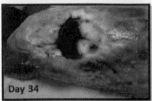
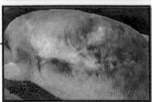

FIG. 8.13 DFU.

Diabetic Foot Ulcer

Year: 2018

Age and Sex: 72, M

Wound site: Left foot

Duration of treatment: 75 days

Cause of wound: Neuroischemic DFU after surgical debridement.

Treatment: Nano colloidal silver solution was used for wound disinfection. Sodium alginate was used for autolytic debridement. After removal of necrotic tissue, treatment was continued with chitosan (gel and powder) and calcium alginate for tissue regeneration.

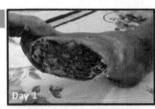
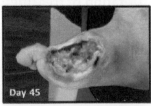
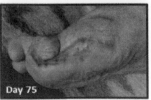

FIG. 8.14 DFU.

Diabetic Foot Ulcer

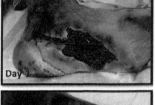
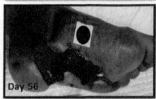
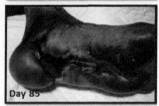

Year: 2018

Age and Sex: 56, M

Wound site: Left foot

Duration of treatment: 85 days

Cause of wound: Neuropathic ulcer with exposed bone and tendon.

Treatment: Nano colloidal silver solution was used for wound disinfection. Sodium alginate and chitosan powder were used for autolytic debridement and tissue regeneration respectively. After removal of necrotic tissue, treatment was continued with calcium alginate.

FIG. 8.15 DFU.

Diabetic Foot Ulcer

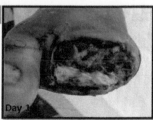
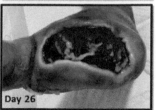
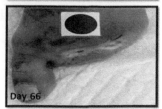

Year: 2018

Age and Sex: 58, M

Wound site: Left toes

Duration of treatment: 66 days

Cause of wound: Necrotic wound after surgical amputation.

Treatment: Nano colloidal silver solution was used for wound disinfection. Sodium alginate was used for autolytic debridement. After removal of necrotic tissue, treatment was continued with chitosan gel and calcium alginate.

FIG. 8.16 DFU.

Diabetic Foot Ulcer

Year: 2018

Age and Sex: 51, M

Wound site: Right toes

Duration of treatment: 24 days

Cause of wound: Neuroischemia.

Treatment: Nano colloidal silver solution was used for wound disinfection. Sodium alginate and chitosan gel were used for autolytic debridement and tissue regeneration, respectively.

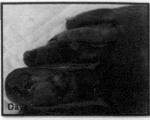
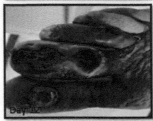
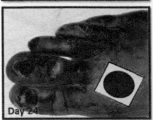
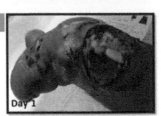

FIG. 8.17 DFU.

Diabetic Foot Ulcer

Year: 2018

Age and Sex: 48, M

Wound site: Left foot

Duration of treatment: 60 days

Cause of wound: Neuroischemia.

Treatment: Nano colloidal silver solution was used for wound disinfection. Sodium alginate and chitosan gel were used for autolytic debridement and tissue regeneration, respectively.

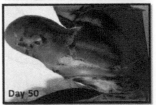
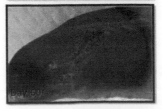

FIG. 8.18 DFU.

Diabetic Foot Ulcer

Year: 2018

Age and Sex: 33, M

Wound site: Right sole

Duration of treatment: 88 days

Cause of wound: Chronic ulcer after surgical debridement.

Treatment: Nano colloidal silver solution was used for wound disinfection. Sodium alginate and chitosan powder were used for autolytic debridement and tissue regeneration respectively. After removal of necrotic tissue, treatment was continued with calcium alginate.

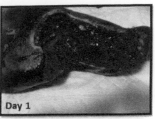
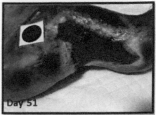
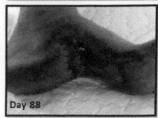
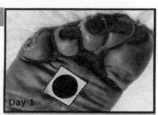

FIG. 8.19 DFU.

Diabetic Foot Ulcer

Year: 2018

Age and Sex: 81, M

Wound site: Right toes

Duration of treatment: 15 days

Cause of wound: Ischemia.

Treatment: Nano colloidal silver solution was used for wound disinfection. Sodium alginate was used for autolytic debridement. After removal of necrotic tissue, treatment was continued with chitosan gel.

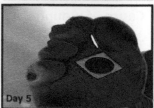
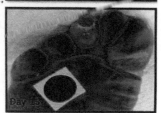

FIG. 8.20 DFU.

Diabetic Foot Ulcer

Year: 2018

Age and Sex: 57, F

Wound site: Right big toe

Duration of treatment: 28 days

Cause of wound: Ischemia.

Treatment: Nano colloidal silver solution was used for wound disinfection. Sodium alginate was used for autolytic debridement. After removal of necrotic tissue, treatment was continued with chitosan gel.

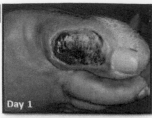
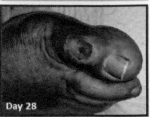
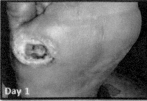

FIG. 8.21 DFU.

Diabetic Foot Ulcer

Year: 2018

Age and Sex: 50, M

Wound site: Right foot

Duration of treatment: 40 days

Cause of wound: Neuropathic ulcer, malum perforans pedis.

Treatment: Nano colloidal silver solution was used for wound disinfection. After sharp debridement of wound edges, sodium alginate and chitosan (powder and gel) were used for autolytic debridement and tissue regeneration, respectively.

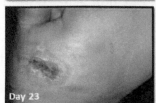
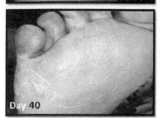

FIG. 8.22 DFU.

Diabetic Foot Ulcer

Year: 2018

Age and Sex: 60, M

Wound site: Right foot

Duration of treatment: 43 days

Cause of wound: Neuropathic ulcer.

Treatment: Nano colloidal silver solution was used for wound disinfection. After sharp debridement of indurated edges, sodium alginate was used for autolytic debridement. Calcium alginate and chitosan gel were used for tissue regeneration.

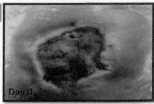
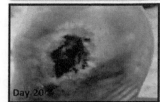
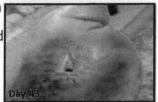

FIG. 8.23 DFU.

Diabetic Foot Ulcer

Year: 2017

Age and Sex: 68, M

Wound site: Right foot

Duration of treatment: 80 days

Cause of wound: Surgical amputation of fifth toe.

Treatment: Nano colloidal silver solution was used for wound disinfection. Sodium alginate and chitosan (powder and gel) were used for autolytic debridement and tissue regeneration, respectively.

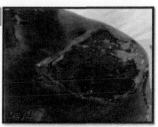
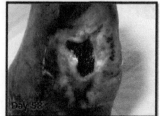
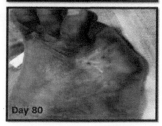

FIG. 8.24 DFU.

Diabetic Foot Ulcer

Year: 2017

Age and Sex: 70, M

Wound site: Left foot

Duration of treatment: 75 days

Cause of wound: Wound infection after amputation.

Treatment: Nano colloidal silver solution was used for wound disinfection. After autolytic debridement with sodium alginate, calcium alginate and chitosan gel were used for tissue regeneration.

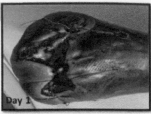
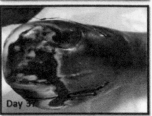
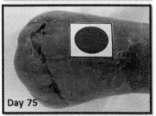

FIG. 8.25 DFU.

Diabetic Foot Ulcer

Year: 2017

Age and Sex: 60, F

Wound site: Right heel

Duration of treatment: 59 days

Cause of wound: Neuropathic ulcer.

Treatment: Nano colloidal silver solution was used for wound disinfection. After sharp removal of blister, treatment was continued with chitosan (powder and gel) and calcium alginate.

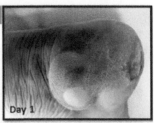
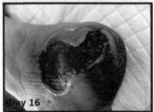
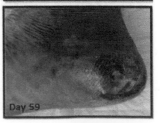

FIG. 8.26 DFU.

Diabetic Foot Ulcer

Year: 2017

Age and Sex: 68, M

Wound site: Right foot

Duration of treatment: 69 days

Cause of wound: Wound infection after amputation of fourth and fifth toes.

Treatment: Nano colloidal silver solution was used for wound disinfection. Sodium alginate was used for autolytic debridement. Afterwards calcium alginate and chitosan gel were used for tissue regeneration.

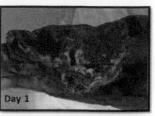
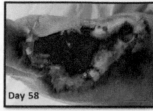
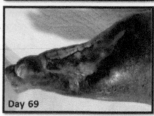

FIG. 8.27 DFU.

Diabetic Foot Ulcer

Year: 2017

Age and Sex: 58, M

Wound site: Right leg

Duration of treatment: 59 days

Cause of wound: Wound infection after surgical amputation.

Treatment: Nano colloidal silver solution was used for wound disinfection. Sodium alginate and chitosan (powder and gel) were used for autolytic debridement and tissue regeneration, respectively.

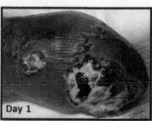
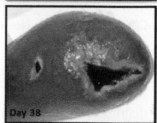
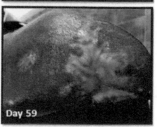

FIG. 8.28 DFU.

Diabetic Foot Ulcer

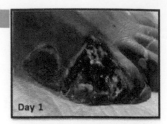

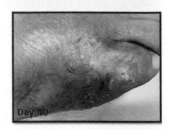

Year: 2017

Age and Sex: 50, F

Wound site: Right foot

Duration of treatment: 40 days

Cause of wound: Ischemia.

Treatment: Nano colloidal silver solution was used for wound disinfection. After removal of necrotic and slough tissue with sodium alginate, treatment was continued with chitosan gel.

FIG. 8.29 DFU.

Diabetic Foot Ulcer

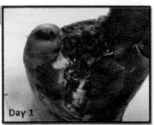

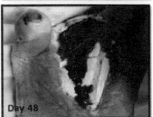

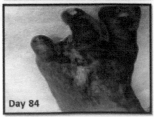

Year: 2017

Age and Sex: 54, F

Wound site: Left foot

Duration of treatment: 84 days

Cause of wound: Neuroishcemic ulcer after amputation of third and fourth toes.

Treatment: Nano colloidal silver solution was used for wound disinfection. Sodium alginate was used for autolytic debridement. After removal of necrotic tissue, treatment was continued with chitosan (powder and gel) and calcium alginate.

FIG. 8.30 DFU.

Diabetic Foot Ulcer

Year: 2017

Age and Sex: 63, M

Wound site: Right big toe

Duration of treatment: 22 days

Cause of wound: Neuropathic ulcer.

Treatment: Nano colloidal silver solution was used for wound disinfection. Sodium alginate and chitosan gel were used for autolytic debridement and tissue regeneration, respectively.

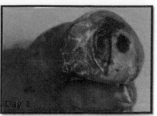
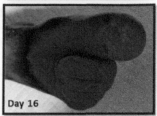
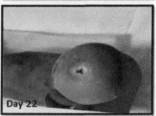

FIG. 8.31 DFU.

Diabetic Foot Ulcer

Year: 2017

Age and Sex: 79, M

Wound site: Right foot

Duration of treatment: 8 days

Cause of wound: Contact burn in a neuropathic foot.

Treatment: Nano colloidal silver solution was used for wound disinfection. Chitosan gel was applied for tissue regeneration.

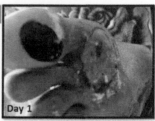
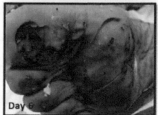
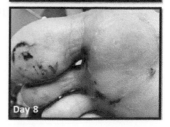

FIG. 8.32 DFU.

Diabetic Foot Ulcer

Year: 2017

Age and Sex: 63, M

Wound site: Left foot

Duration of treatment: 48 days

Cause of wound: Neuropathic ulcer, malum perforans pedis.

Treatment: Nano colloidal silver solution was used for wound disinfection. Sodium alginate and chitosan gel were used for autolytic debridement and tissue regeneration, respectively.

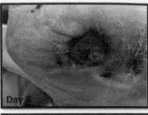
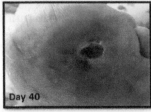
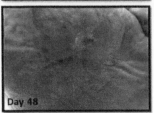

FIG. 8.33 DFU.

Diabetic Foot Ulcer

Year: 2017

Age and Sex: 45, F

Wound site: Left Dorsum

Duration of treatment: 49 days

Cause of wound: Ischemic ulcer 30 days after removal of blister.

Treatment: Nano colloidal silver solution was used for wound disinfection. After autolytic debridement with sodium alginate, treatment was continued with chitosan gel and powder.

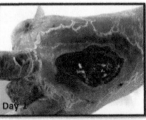
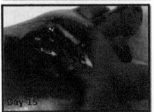
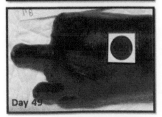

FIG. 8.34 DFU.

Diabetic Foot Ulcer

Year: 2016

Age and Sex: 26, F

Wound site: Right foot

Duration of treatment: 15 days

Cause of wound: Auto-amputation of fifth toe.

Treatment: Nano colloidal silver solution was used for wound disinfection. Sodium alginate and chitosan were used for autolytic debridement and tissue regeneration, respectively.

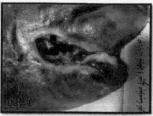
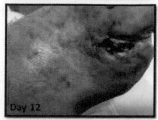
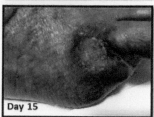

FIG. 8.35 DFU.

Diabetic Foot Ulcer

Year: 2016

Age and Sex: 59, M

Wound site: Right foot

Duration of treatment: 41 days

Cause of wound: Ischemia.

Treatment: Nano colloidal silver solution was used for wound disinfection. Sodium alginate and chitosan gel were used for autolytic debridement and tissue regeneration, respectively.

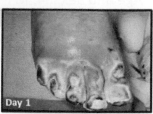
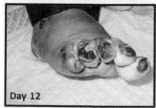
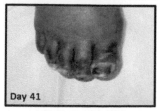

FIG. 8.36 DFU.

Diabetic Foot Ulcer

Year: 2014

Age and Sex: 63, F

Wound site: Left sole

Duration of treatment: 10 days

Cause of wound: Contact burn in a neuropathic foot.

Treatment: Nano colloidal silver solution was used for wound disinfection. Chitosan gel was applied for tissue regeneration.

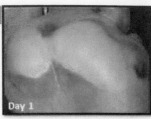

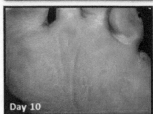

FIG. 8.37 DFU.

Diabetic Foot Ulcer

Year: 2014

Age and Sex: 34, M

Wound site: Left foot

Duration of treatment: 46 days

Cause of wound: Neuroischemia.

Treatment: Nano colloidal silver solution was used for wound disinfection. After sharp debridement of indurated wound edge and yellow callus tissue, treatment was continued with chitosan powder and gel.

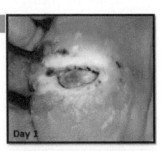

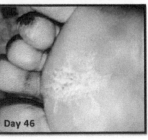

FIG. 8.38 DFU.

Diabetic Foot Ulcer

Year: 2014

Age and Sex: 70, M

Wound site: Right big toe

Duration of treatment: 30 days

Cause of wound: Ischemia.

Treatment: Nano colloidal silver solution was used for wound disinfection. Sodium alginate and chitosan gel were used for autolytic debridement and tissue regeneration, respectively.

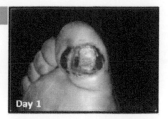
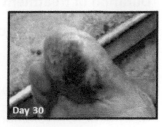

FIG. 8.39 DFU.

Diabetic Foot Ulcer

Year: 2010

Age and Sex: 51, M

Wound site: Left foot

Duration of treatment: 60 days

Cause of wound: Wound dehiscence after amputation of fifth toe.

Treatment: Nano colloidal silver solution was used for wound disinfection. Sodium alginate and chitosan (powder and gel) were used for autolytic debridement and tissue regeneration, respectively.

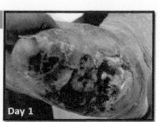
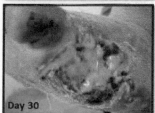
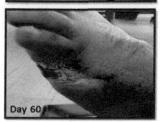

FIG. 8.40 DFU.

Diabetic Foot Ulcer

Year: 2009

Age and Sex: 54, F

Wound site: Right big toe

Duration of treatment: 50 days

Cause of wound: 18-years history of diabetes with neuroischemic ulcer.

Treatment: Nano colloidal silver solution was used for wound disinfection. After sharp debridement of wound edges, sodium alginate was used for softening the fibrotic tissue and chitosan powder was applied for tissue regeneration.

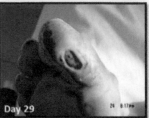
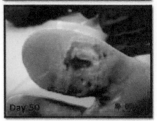
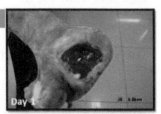

FIG. 8.41 DFU.

Diabetic Foot Ulcer

Year: 2009

Age and Sex: 68, M

Wound site: Right foot

Duration of treatment: 40 days

Cause of wound: Surgical amputation (20-years history of diabetes).

Treatment: Nano colloidal silver solution was used for wound disinfection. Chitosan powder and gel were applied for tissue regeneration.

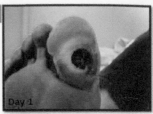
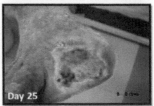
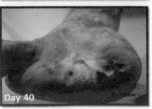

FIG. 8.42 DFU.

Diabetic Foot Ulcer

Year: 2009

Age and Sex: 73, M

Wound site: Left foot

Duration of treatment: 50 days

Cause of wound: Surgical amputation.

Treatment: Nano colloidal silver solution was used for wound disinfection. After sharp debridement of wound edge, sodium alginate and chitosan powder were used for autolytic debridement and tissue regeneration, respectively.

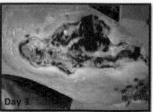
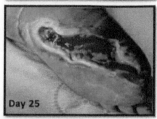
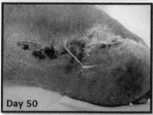

FIG. 8.43 DFU.

Diabetic Foot Ulcer

Year: 2006

Age and Sex: 65, M

Wound site: Right foot

Duration of treatment: 58 days

Cause of wound: Ischemia.

Treatment: Nano colloidal silver solution was used for wound disinfection. Sodium alginate was used for autolytic debridement along with sharp debridement. After removal of necrotic tissue, treatment was continued with chitosan powder and gel.

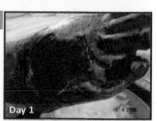
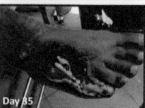
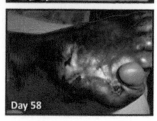

FIG. 8.44 DFU.

CHAPTER 9

Burn Wounds

Burn is one of the major types of acute wound, caused by thermal, chemical, or electrical contact, radiation, etc., which results in tissue damage. Burn wounds are highly variable based on the severity and affected tissue type. Following the burn injury, a systemic response occurs and alters the normal physiological state of the body [101].

There are various types of burns depending on the causative agent:
- Physical
- Thermal burns
  - By dry heat
  - By wet heat
- Electrical burns
- Radiation burns
- Laser burns
- Chemical (acid burns, alkali burns, others) [102].

TYPES OF BURN

Burn wounds can be classified based on severity, type of involved tissues, and depth, as follows:
- **First-degree burn:** A localized injury causes damage to the epidermis, characterized by localized pain, edema, and erythema, and usually without blister.

  First-degree burn does not disrupt the barrier function of the skin and is not a life threatening condition (Fig. 9.1).
- **Second-degree burn:** Involves the epidermis and variable thickness of the dermis. It is subclassified as follows:
  - **Superficial second-degree burn:** In which the epidermis and papillary dermis are damaged. It is characterized by pain, early blister formation, exposed nerve endings, lost barrier function of the skin, and inflammation (Fig. 9.2).
  - **Deep second-degree burn:** Involves epidermis, papillary dermis, and deep reticular dermis. It is characterized by blister formation, mild edema, pain, intact hair follicle, and extensive disruption of sensory nerves (Fig. 9.3).
- **Third-degree burn or full-thickness burn:** Involves the epidermis, the dermis, and the hypodermis. It may extend to the underlying muscle, bone, and interstitial tissues. It is characterized by dry dark leather-like appearance without blister. It is usually painless because of irreversible damage of nerves [101–103] (Fig. 9.4).

Fig. 9.5 shows the different degrees of burn wound schematically.

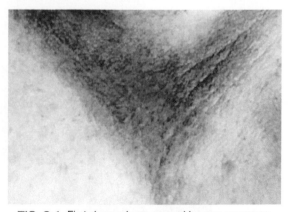

FIG. 9.1 First-degree burn caused by sun exposure.

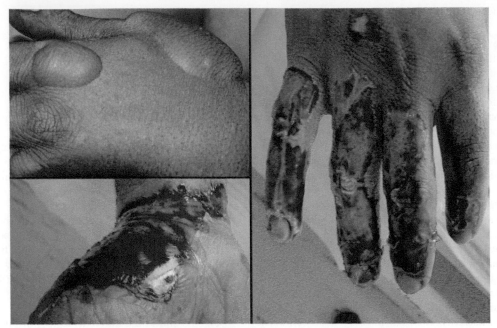

FIG. 9.2 Blisters formed in a superficial second-degree wound.

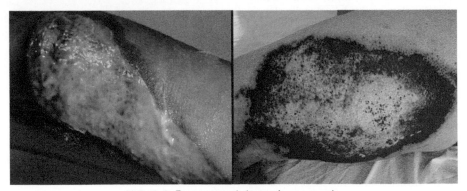

FIG. 9.3 Deep second-degree burn wounds.

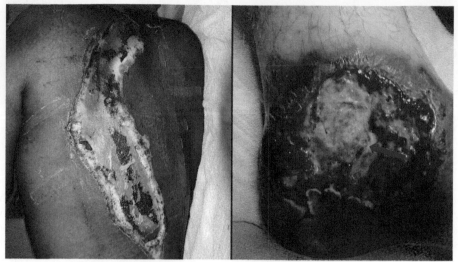

FIG. 9.4 Third-degree burn wounds.

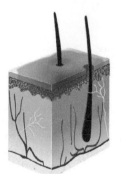 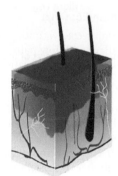 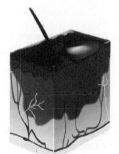 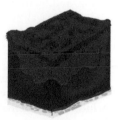

First-degree burn   Superficial second-degree burn   Deep second-degree burn   Third-degree burn

FIG. 9.5 Degrees of burn wound.

RULE OF NINES

The rule of nines, also known as Wallace rule of nines, is a practical technique for calculating the percentage of total body surface area (TBSA) in patients with partial-thickness or full-thickness burns. Patients with second-degree and third-degree burns lose massive fluid and suffer from dehydration due to the damage or removal of the skin as barrier. Hence, it is crucial to specify the wound severity and fluid resuscitation requirements for better wound care management.

Moreover, the percentage in rule of nines may be altered by the patient's body mass index (BMI) and age.

According to the rule of nines, each part of the body has a certain percentage of nine or a multiple of nine (Fig. 9.6) [104].

Wound Care Management and Early Treatment for Burn Wounds

1. Estimate degree of burn (first, second, or third)
2. Estimate the extent of burn based on rule of nines

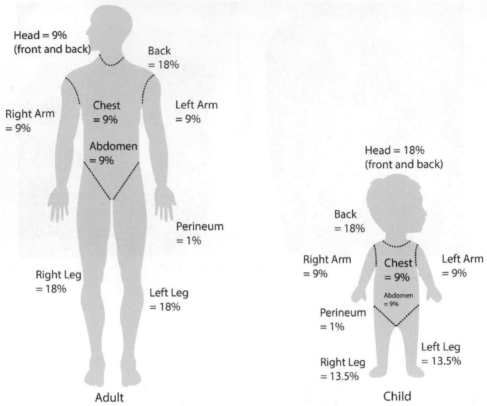

FIG. 9.6 Rule of nines refers a certain percentage to each part of the body.

3. According to the burn severity patient should be hospitalized and receives appropriate medical care, including debridement, ulcer bed preparation, and skin grafts.

4. Apply antiseptic solutions and provide appropriate wound dressing for home care.

Case Reports

Figs. 9.7 to 9.25 show the treatment process for burn wounds.

Burn Wound

Year: 2018

Age and Sex: 31, F

Wound site: Face

Duration of treatment: 15 days

Cause of wound: Superficial second-degree burn wound caused by acid (chemical burn).

Treatment: Nano colloidal silver solution was used for wound disinfection. Chitosan gel was used for tissue regeneration.

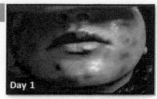
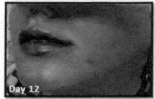
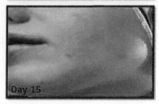

FIG. 9.7 Burn.

Burn Wound

Year: 2018

Age and Sex: 13, M

Wound site: Left leg

Duration of treatment: 19 days

Cause of wound: Deep second-degree burn wound caused by flame.

Treatment: Nano colloidal silver solution was used for wound disinfection. Sodium alginate and chitosan gel were used for autolytic debridement and tissue regeneration, respectively.

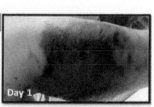
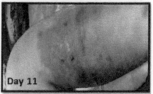
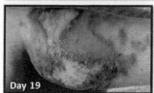

FIG. 9.8 Burn.

Burn Wound

Year: 2017

Age and Sex: 35, M

Wound site: Right hand

Duration of treatment: 15 days

Cause of wound: Deep second-degree burn wound caused by hot coal.

Treatment: Nano colloidal silver solution was used for wound disinfection. Chitosan gel was used for tissue regeneration.

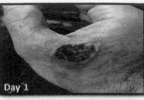
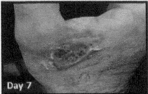
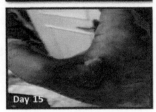

FIG. 9.9　Burn.

Burn Wound

Year: 2016

Age and Sex: 7 months, M

Wound site: Face

Duration of treatment: 28 days

Cause of wound: Deep second-degree burn wound caused by hot coal.

Treatment: Nano colloidal silver solution was used for wound disinfection. Sodium alginate and chitosan gel were used for autolytic debridement and tissue regeneration, respectively.

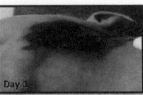
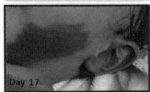
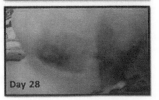

FIG. 9.10　Burn.

Burn Wound

Year: 2015

Age and Sex: 56, M

Wound site: Left Foot

Duration of treatment: 37 days

Cause of wound: Third-degree burn wound caused by gasoline.

Treatment: Nano colloidal silver solution was used for wound disinfection. Sodium alginate was used for autolytic removal of yellow slough tissue and calcium alginate and chitosan gel were applied for tissue regeneration.

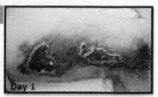
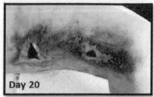
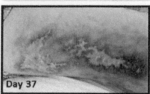

FIG. 9.11 Burn.

Burn Wound

Year: 2015

Age and Sex: 64, M

Wound site: Right Leg

Duration of treatment: 26 days

Cause of wound: Deep second-degree burn wound caused by radiotherapy.

Treatment: Nano colloidal silver solution was used for wound disinfection. Sodium alginate and chitosan gel were used for autolytic debridement and tissue regeneration.

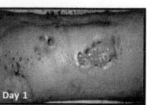
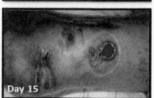
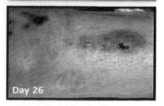

FIG. 9.12 Burn.

Burn Wound

Year: 2015

Age and Sex: 56, M

Wound site: Left Foot

Duration of treatment: 60 days

Cause of wound: Third-degree burn wound caused by gasoline.

Treatment: Nano colloidal silver solution was used for wound disinfection. Sodium alginate was applied for autolytic removal of yellow slough tissue and calcium alginate and chitosan gel were used for tissue regeneration.

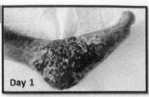
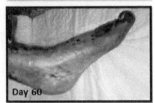
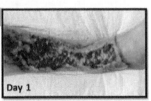
Day 1

Day 30

Day 60

FIG. 9.13 Burn.

Burn Wound

Year: 2015

Age and Sex: 56, M

Wound site: Right Leg

Duration of treatment: 60 days

Cause of wound: Third-degree burn wound caused by gasoline.

Treatment: Nano colloidal silver solution was used for wound disinfection. Sodium alginate was used for autolytic removal of yellow slough tissue and calcium alginate and chitosan gel were applied for tissue regeneration.

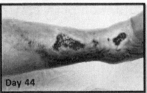
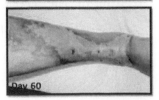
Day 1

Day 44

Day 60

FIG. 9.14 Burn.

Burn Wound

Year: 2014

Age and Sex: 5, F

Wound site: Face

Duration of treatment: 30 days

Cause of wound: Deep second-degree burn wound caused by a hot object.

Treatment: Nano colloidal silver solution was used for wound disinfection. Sodium alginate and chitosan gel were used for autolytic debridement and tissue regeneration, respectively.

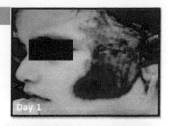
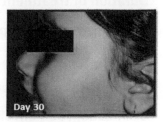

FIG. 9.15 Burn.

Burn Wound

Year: 2014

Age and Sex: 49, M

Wound site: Right foot

Duration of treatment: 34 days

Cause of wound: Deep second-degree burn wound caused by boiling water.

Treatment: Nano colloidal silver solution was used for wound disinfection. Sodium alginate was used for autolytic removal of yellow slough tissue and calcium alginate was applied for tissue regeneration.

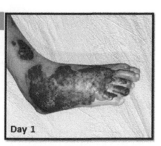
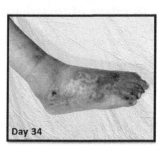

FIG. 9.16 Burn.

Burn Wound

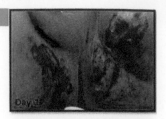

Year: 2014

Age and Sex: 49, M

Wound site: Groin

Duration of treatment: 21 days

Cause of wound: Deep second-degree burn wound with hot water.

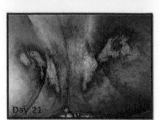

Treatment: Nano colloidal silver solution was used for wound disinfection. Sodium alginate was used for autolytic removal of yellow slough tissue and calcium alginate was applied for tissue regeneration.

FIG. 9.17 Burn.

Burn Wound

Year: 2014

Age and Sex: 46, M

Wound site: Right foot

Duration of treatment: 40 days

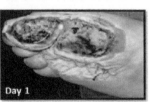

Cause of wound: Third-degree burn wound caused by a hot object.

Treatment: Nano colloidal silver solution was used for wound disinfection. Sodium alginate was used for autolytic debridement then treatment was continued with chitosan gel.

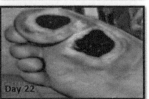

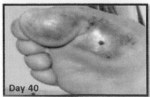

FIG. 9.18 Burn.

Burn Wound

Year: 2014

Age and Sex: 1, F

Wound site: Left shoulder

Duration of treatment: 35 days

Cause of wound: Deep second-degree burn wound caused by boiling milk.

Treatment: Nano colloidal silver solution was used for wound disinfection. Sodium alginate and chitosan gel were applied for autolytic debridement and tissue regeneration, respectively.

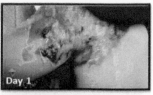
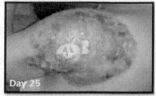
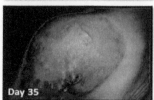

FIG. 9.19 Burn.

Burn Wound

Year: 2006

Age and Sex: 26, F

Wound site: Abdominal region

Duration of treatment: 28 days

Cause of wound: Deep second-degree burn wound caused by boiling water.

Treatment: Nano colloidal silver solution was used for wound disinfection. Sodium alginate and chitosan were used for autolytic debridement and tissue regeneration, respectively.

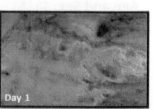
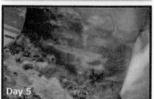
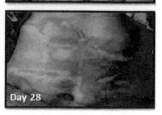

FIG. 9.20 Burn.

Burn Wound

Year: 2006

Age and Sex: 53, F

Wound site: Left big toe

Duration of treatment: 17 days

Cause of wound: Deep second-degree burn wound caused by a hot object.

Treatment: Nano colloidal silver solution was used for wound disinfection. Chitosan gel was used for tissue regeneration.

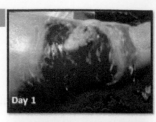
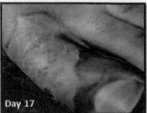

FIG. 9.21 Burn.

Burn Wound

Year: 2006

Age and Sex: 41, M

Wound site: Dorsum of right hand

Duration of treatment: 7 days

Cause of wound: Deep second-degree burn wound caused by boiling water.

Treatment: Nano colloidal silver solution was used for wound disinfection. Chitosan gel was used for tissue regeneration.

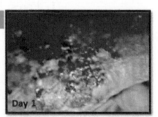
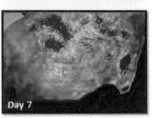

FIG. 9.22 Burn.

Burn Wound

Year: 2006

Age and Sex: 22, M

Wound site: Right thigh

Duration of treatment: 15 days

Cause of wound: Deep second-degree burn wound caused by a hot object.

Treatment: Nano colloidal silver solution was used for wound disinfection. Sodium alginate and chitosan gel were used for autolytic debridement and tissue regeneration, respectively.

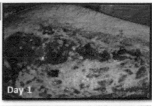
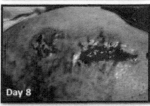
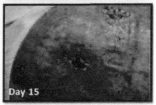

FIG. 9.23 Burn.

Burn Wound

Year: 2005

Age and Sex: 23, M

Wound site: Face

Duration of treatment: 6 days

Cause of wound: Superficial second-degree burn wound caused by flame.

Treatment: Nano colloidal silver solution was used for wound disinfection. Chitosan gel was used for tissue regeneration.

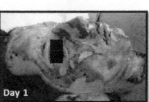
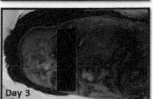
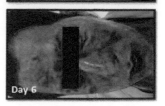

FIG. 9.24 Burn.

Burn Wound

Year: 2005

Age and Sex: 21, M

Wound site: Right side of face and ear

Duration of treatment: 4 days

Cause of wound: Superficial second-degree burn wound caused by boiling water.

Treatment: Nano colloidal silver solution was used for wound disinfection. Chitosan gel was used for tissue regeneration.

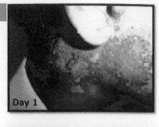
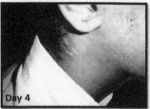

FIG. 9.25 Burn.

CHAPTER 10

Vascular Ulcers

Commonly, a large number of men older than 45 and women older than 55, and patients with a family history of premature atherosclerotic disease, experience peripheral vascular disease in their life. Multiple factors such as smoking, diabetes, obesity, high blood pressure, high cholesterol, and high levels of homocysteine; increases the risk of developing peripheral vascular disease[105].

The human body vascular system consists of veins, arteries, and lymphatic vessels, in which vascular ulcer may occur. Fig. 10.1 illustrates the gradual development of vascular ulcers, and Fig. 10.2 shows the different types of vascular ulcers.

VENOUS ULCERS

Venous ulcers are open sores that occur due to inappropriate function of venous valves, sustained venous hypertension, and usually appear between the knee and the ankle.

Venous ulcers are the most common vascular ulcers and difficult to heal. The ulcer may be superficial with minimal to severe serous discharge and granulation tissue in wound bed.

Pain may be present especially when foot is in dependent position [106] (Fig. 10.3).

ARTERIAL ULCERS

Arterial ulcers usually occur in lower extremities below the ankles, particularly in the tips of toes following the insufficient arterial blood supply. These ulcers progress more rapidly by aging, smoking, atherosclerotic diseases, diabetes, hypertension, dyslipidemia, family history, or obesity. Arterial ulcers are characterized by pain especially at night [105,106] (Fig. 10.4).

LYMPHATIC ULCERS

Lymphedema is a progressive condition that causes by accumulation of lymphatic fluid in the interstitial space of body tissue due to obstruction in the lymphatic system. Lymphedema skin ulcers are superficial with round edges and shallow moist bed. The surrounding skin is usually fibrotic and thickened by

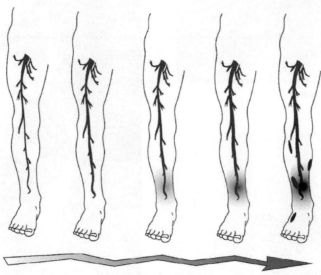

Time (months to years)

FIG. 10.1 Schematic view of vascular ulcers progression against time.

Atlas of Wound Healing. https://doi.org/10.1016/B978-0-323-67968-8.00010-0

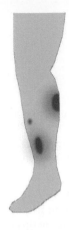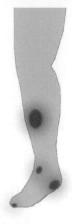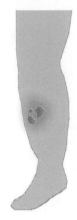

Venus ulcers   Arterial ulcers   Lymphatic ulcers and edema

FIG. 10.2 Different types of vascular ulcers.

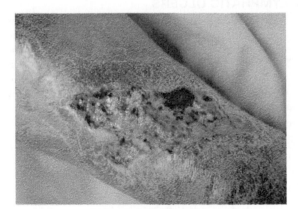

FIG. 10.3 Venous ulcer.

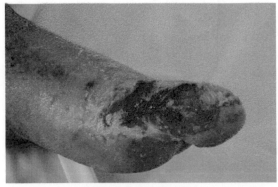

FIG. 10.4 Arterial ulcer.

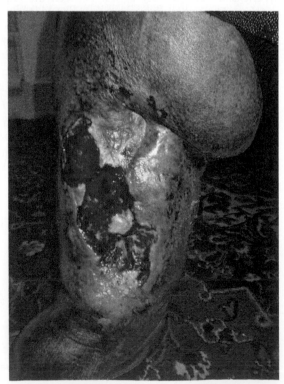

FIG. 10.5 Lymphatic ulcer.

edema. However, the ulcer development in chronic lymphedema is less frequent than venous ulcers or arterial ulcers; but it is more complicated [107,108] (Fig. 10.5).

The clinical characteristics of vascular ulcers are presented in Table 10.1.

Wound Care Management and Early Treatment for Vascular Ulcers

1. Assess the arterial pulses to check the blood flow of lower extremity (femoral, popliteal, posterior tibial, and dorsalis pedis pulses) (Fig. 10.6).

2. Ask patient to quit smoking.
3. Get vascular consult to treat underlying vascular diseases (e.g., bypass, angioplasty, etc.)
4. In case of ischemia or insufficient blood supply, mechanical debridement must be avoided.
5. In case of infection, start antibiotic administration under medical supervision.
6. In case of necrotic tissue formation, apply sharp or autolytic debridement.
7. Apply antiseptic solutions and provide appropriate wound dressing.

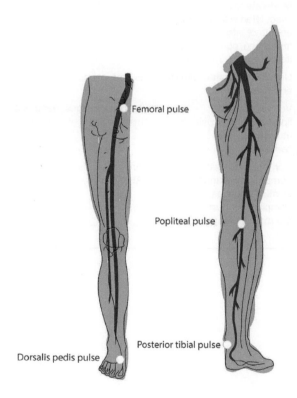

FIG. 10.6 Arterial pulse points.

TABLE 10.1
Clinical Characteristics of Different Types of Vascular Ulcer [105,106]

	Venous	Arterial	Lymphatic
Etiology	Varicosis, deep vein thrombosis, venous insufficiency	Family history of peripheral arterial disease, claudication, rest pain	Lymphedema
Common site	Between the knee and the ankle	Below the ankle and tip of toes, corners of nail beds on toes, over bony prominences, and between toes	Arms, legs, and ankle area
Edges	Irregular sloping edges	Punched-out edges	Sloping edges
Wound bed and surrounding skin	Superficial with granulation tissue with slough tissue	Slough and necrotic tissue	Surrounding skin is usually firm, fibrotic, and thickened by edema
Exudate level	Usually high	Usually low	Medium to high
Pain	Moderate to no pain unless associated with extreme edema or infection (throbbing, burning, and itchy)	Very painful (sharp and hurting), even without infection	Painful
Edema	Usually associated with limb edema	Edema not common	Usually associated with edema
Associated features	Venous eczema, lipodermatosclerosis, atrophy blanche, hemosiderosis	Trophic changes; gangrene may be occur	Cellulitis (tissue inflammation) may occur
Treatment	Compression using compression bandages, elastic bandages, compression pumps, etc. is the main therapy.	Arterial bypass Angioplasty	Limb elevation and using compression pump for reducing edema Massage therapy for reducing edema as well as circulation improving

Case Reports

Figs. 10.7 to 10.14 show the treatment process for vascular ulcers.

Vascular Ulcer

Year: 2018

Age and Sex: 85, M

Wound site: Left leg

Duration of treatment: 50 days

Cause of wound: Venous ulcer.

Treatment: Nano colloidal silver solution was used for wound disinfection. Sodium alginate and chitosan gel were applied for autolytic removal of yellow slough tissue and tissue regeneration, respectively.

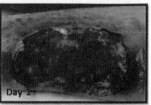
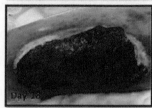
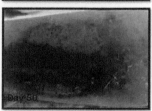

FIG. 10.7 Vascular ulcer.

Vascular Ulcer

Year: 2018

Age and Sex: 64, F

Wound site: Left foot

Duration of treatment: 47 days

Cause of wound: Arterial ulcer (addicted and heavy smoker).

Treatment: Nano colloidal silver solution was used for wound disinfection. Sodium alginate was used for autolytic debridement. After removal of necrotic tissue, treatment was continued with chitosan gel and calcium alginate.

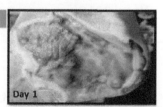
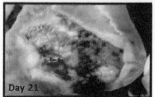
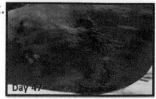

FIG. 10.8 Vascular ulcer.

Vascular Ulcer

Year: 2017

Age and Sex: 43, F

Wound site: Right leg

Duration of treatment: 18 days

Cause of wound: A venous ulcer caused by vascular and lymphatic insufficiency in a heavy smoker patient.

Treatment: Nano colloidal silver solution was used for wound disinfection. Sodium alginate was used for autolytic debridement. After removal of necrotic tissue, treatment was continued with chitosan gel. Patient expired during treatment.

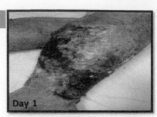
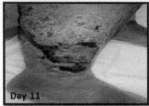
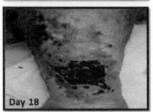

FIG. 10.9 Vascular ulcer.

Vascular Ulcer

Year: 2016

Age and Sex: 57, M

Wound site: Right leg

Duration of treatment: 60 days

Cause of wound: Vascular and lymphatic insufficiency.

Treatment: Nano colloidal silver solution was used for wound disinfection. Chitosan gel was applied for tissue regeneration.

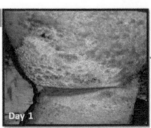
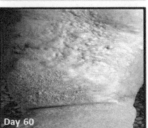

FIG. 10.10 Vascular ulcer.

Vascular Ulcer

Year: 2015

Age and Sex: 46, M

Wound site: Right hand

Duration of treatment: 51 days

Cause of wound: Patient is a victim of chemical warfare suffering from vascular insufficiency.

Treatment: Nano colloidal silver solution was used for wound disinfection. Sodium alginate and chitosan were used for autolytic debridement and tissue regeneration, respectively.

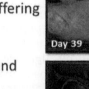
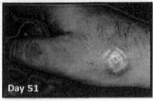
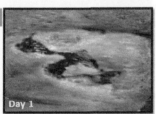

FIG. 10.11 Vascular ulcer.

Vascular Ulcer

Year: 2015

Age and Sex: 68, F

Wound site: Right leg

Duration of treatment: 60 days

Cause of wound: Vascular and lymphatic insufficiency.

Treatment: Nano colloidal silver solution was used for wound disinfection. Sodium alginate was applied for autolytic removal of yellow slough tissue. Calcium alginate and chitosan gel were applied for tissue regeneration.

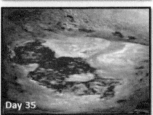
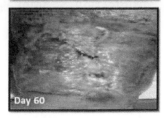

FIG. 10.12 Vascular ulcer.

Vascular Ulcer

Year: 2015

Age and Sex: 68, F

Wound site: Left leg

Duration of treatment: 60 days

Cause of wound: Vascular and lymphatic insufficiency.

Treatment: Nano colloidal silver solution was used for wound disinfection. Sodium alginate was applied for autolytic removal of yellow slough tissue. Calcium alginate and chitosan gel were applied for tissue regeneration.

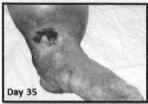
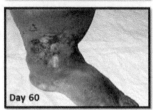
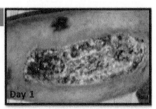

FIG. 10.13 Vascular ulcer.

Vascular Ulcer

Year: 2015

Age and Sex: 46, M

Wound site: Left leg

Duration of treatment: 65 days

Cause of wound: Patient is a victim of chemical warfare suffering from vascular insufficiency.

Treatment: Nano colloidal silver solution was used for wound disinfection. Sodium alginate and chitosan were used for autolytic debridement and tissue regeneration, respectively.

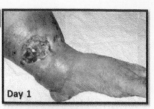
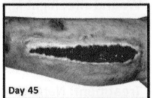
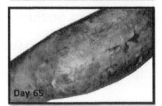

FIG. 10.14 Vascular ulcer.

CHAPTER 11

Traumatic Wounds

Traumatic wounds are acute or newly occurred wounds in various types such as cuts, lacerations, abrasions, scratches, or punctures. Fig. 11.1 shows the traumatic wound schematically.

CUT WOUNDS

A cut wound is usually caused by a sharp object (e.g., knife) with a blunt additional force, in which underlying tissues may be involved depending on the wound depth and severity. The wound edges in cuts are sharp, open, and clean, and underlying tissues are visible. In large wounds, primary suturing is needed for better wound closure. Wound should be watched for foreign bodies before wound treatment (Fig. 11.2).

LACERATIONS

Lacerations are known as the skin torn due to a rupture or tear split caused by blunt trauma, in which underlying soft tissues such as muscle or tendon may be damaged. Wound edges in laceration are usually irregular and jaggy. Tissue damage may not be extensive, and primary suturing may be needed, while the wound is typically contaminated by debris and pathogens from the external environment and/or the object that caused the wound [109] (Fig. 11.3).

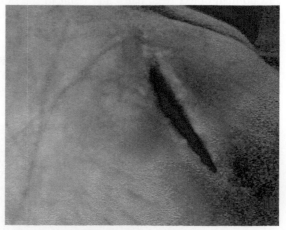

FIG. 11.2 Cut wound.

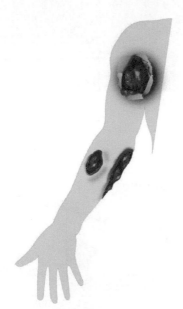

FIG. 11.1 Traumatic wound illustration.

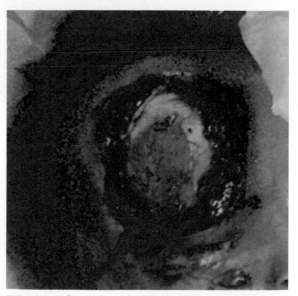

FIG. 11.3 Separation of skin and underlying tissues in which the edges are torn and irregular in a laceration wound caused by accident.

Atlas of Wound Healing. https://doi.org/10.1016/B978-0-323-67968-8.00011-2

CONTUSIONS

Contusions are closed wound caused by blunt or blast trauma. Blood vessels are damaged, and large hematomas under skin or in muscle may form. Extensive contusion may lead to infection [109]. Contusions are characterized by local pain, hematoma, and intact skin (Fig. 11.4).

PUNCTURES

Punctures are deep open wounds caused by a sharp and pointed object (e.g., nail), and result in the skin and/or underlying tissues damage. These wounds seem negligible with raised and round edges (Fig. 11.5).

Punctures cause damage to the muscles, large vessels, parenchymal organs, and nerves. Commonly, puncture wounds may not bleed heavily. Wound healing procedure usually is not going through the normal pathway. It is highly recommended to consider the risk of tetanus and anaerobic infection after a puncture wound.

In most cases of puncture wounds, the foreign body must be assessed and for pulling it out, caution should be taken to avoid damage to the healthy tissues. Fig. 11.6 shows a traumatic wound after the removal of foreign body.

ABRASIONS

Abrasions are superficial wounds caused by frictional scraping forces. Abrasions must be cleansed, and foreign bodies should be removed immediately to avoid the risk of infection. They are usually painful due to many exposed nerve endings, and they proceed in normal wound healing pathway (Fig. 11.7).

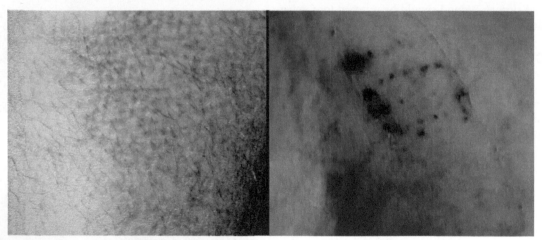

FIG. 11.4 Contusions after trauma.

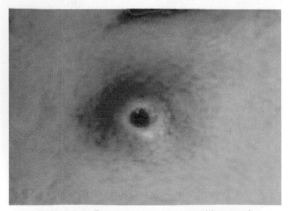

FIG. 11.5 Puncture wound caused by a rod.

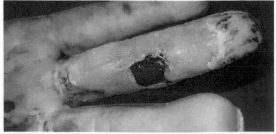

FIG. 11.6 Secondary traumatic wound after removal of a piece of wood from a puncture wound.

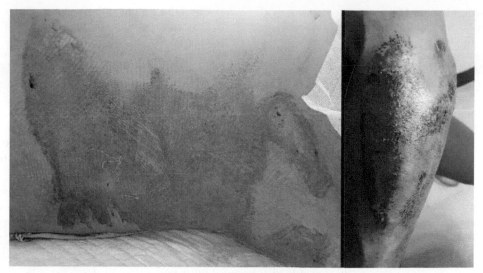

FIG. 11.7 Abrasion wounds.

BITES

Bite wounds are caused by animal or human bite, in which infection may be caused by anaerobic and/or aerobic pathogens from patient's skin and/or animal's mouth, thereby making the treatment difficult [110]. Bite wounds characterized by ragged wounds, crushed tissue, and bone infection may occur. In addition to normal wound treatment, rabies and tetanus injection is needed (Fig. 11.8).

WOUNDS FROM EXPLOSIONS AND GUNSHOT

Wounds caused by gunshot or explosion result in gross skeletal and soft tissue injuries with a deep cavity due to the bullet track. Patient cloths, surrounding tissues, or foreign bodies may be sucked into the wound. Along with ischemia, this contamination may lead to anaerobic infection.

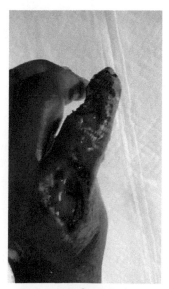

FIG. 11.8 Scorpion bite.

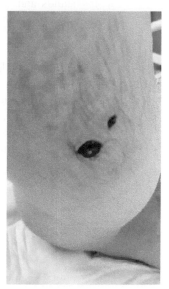

FIG. 11.9 Wound caused by gunshot.

These wounds should be debrided down to the viable tissues, and then should be left open, until formation of healthy granulation tissue (repeated debridement may be necessary). In case of infection after debridement, antibiotic treatment is recommended [109] (Fig. 11.9).

Wound Care Management and Early Treatment for Traumatic Wounds

1. Maintain hemostasis if needed
2. Assess the wound carefully and remove foreign bodies if possible.
3. Clean the wound with isotonic saline or water.
4. Cover the wound with sterile gauze and hospitalize the patient if needed.
5. In case of slough tissue formation, debride the wound until healthy granulation tissue formation.
6. Apply antiseptic solutions and provide appropriate wound dressing.

Case Reports
Figs. 11.10−11.17 show the treatment process for traumatic wounds.

Traumatic Wound

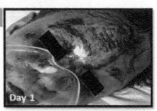

Year: 2018

Age and Sex: 4, F

Wound site: Face

Duration of treatment: 30 days

Cause of wound: Car accident.

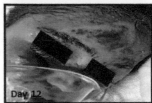

Treatment: Nano colloidal silver solution was used for wound disinfection. Sodium alginate and chitosan gel were used for autolytic debridement and tissue regeneration, respectively.

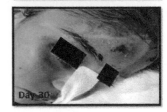

FIG. 11.10 Traumatic wound.

Traumatic Wound

Year: 2018

Age and Sex: 59, M

Wound site: Left foot

Duration of treatment: 62 days

Cause of wound: Traumatic puncture caused by pin, developed to a chronic ulcer in a diabetic patient.

Treatment: Nano colloidal silver solution was used for wound disinfection. Sodium alginate and chitosan (gel and foam) were used for autolytic debridement and tissue regeneration, respectively.

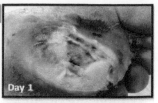
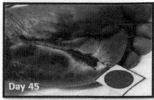
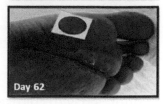

FIG. 11.11 Traumatic wound.

Traumatic Wound

Year: 2018

Age and Sex: 40, M

Wound site: Right leg

Duration of treatment: 15 days

Cause of wound: An avulsion wound caused by a car accident, developed to a chronic ulcer.

Treatment: Nano colloidal silver solution was used for wound disinfection. Sodium alginate was used for autolytic debridement along with sharp debridement, then treatment was continued with chitosan gel and powder.

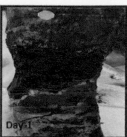
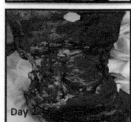
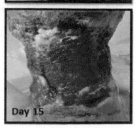

FIG. 11.12 Traumatic wound.

Traumatic Wound

Year: 2017

Age and Sex: 59, M

Wound site: Right leg

Duration of treatment: 28 days

Cause of wound: Abrasion caused by car accident.

Treatment: Nano colloidal silver solution was used for wound disinfection. Sodium alginate was used for autolytic debridement of necrotic tissue. Calcium alginate and chitosan (gel, foam and powder) were applied for tissue regeneration. Treatment was continued with chitosan gel.

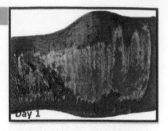
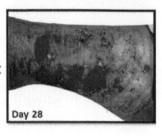

FIG. 11.13 Traumatic wound.

Traumatic Wound

Year: 2017

Age and Sex: 62, F

Wound site: Left foot

Duration of treatment: 50 days

Cause of wound: Car accident, developed to a chronic ulcer.

Treatment: Nano colloidal silver solution was used for wound disinfection. Sodium alginate and chitosan (gel and powder) were used for autolytic debridement and tissue regeneration, respectively.

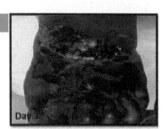
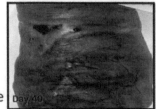
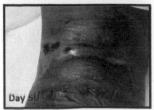

FIG. 11.14 Traumatic wound.

Traumatic Wound

Year: 2010

Age and Sex: 16, F

Wound site: Right heel

Duration of treatment: 40 days

Cause of wound: Avulsion caused by trauma, developed to a chronic ulcer.

Treatment: Nano colloidal silver solution was used for wound disinfection. Sodium alginate was used for autolytic debridement of yellow slough tissue, then treatment was continued with chitosan gel.

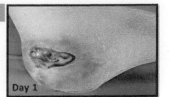
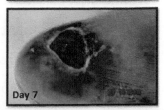
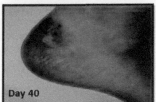

FIG. 11.15 Traumatic wound.

Traumatic Wound

Year: 2005

Age and Sex: 43, F

Wound site: Left leg

Duration of treatment: 72 days

Cause of wound: Car accident developed to a chronic ulcer.

Treatment: Nano colloidal silver solution was used for wound disinfection. Sodium alginate was used for autolytic debridement along with sharp debridement, then treatment was continued with chitosan gel.

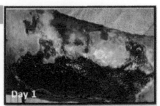
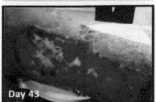
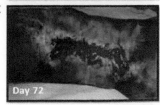

FIG. 11.16 Traumatic wound.

Traumatic Wound

Year: 2005

Age and Sex: 28, M

Wound site: Left foot

Duration of treatment: 67 days

Cause of wound: Avulsion.

Treatment: Nano colloidal silver solution was used for wound disinfection. Sodium alginate and chitosan (gel and powder) were used for autolytic debridement and tissue regeneration, respectively.

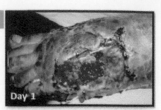
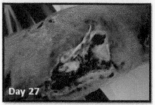
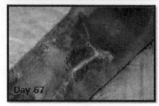

FIG. 11.17 Traumatic wound.

CHAPTER 12

Surgical Incisions

Surgical incisions, as the entry sites to access the body inner organs, cause minimal tissue damage. They are precisely made by sharp instruments in a sterile environment to reduce the risk of infection. Surgical incisions are characterized by sharp wound edges, without severe damage, and usually healed by primary intention. Commonly, the wound margins are approximated by sutures or devices, and in some cases they are left open to heal [109] (Fig. 12.1).

The American College of Surgeons (ACS) classified surgical wounds based on the level of wound contamination, as follows:
1. Clean
2. Clean-contaminated
3. Contaminated
4. Dirty-infected [111].

WOUND DEHISCENCE

Wound dehiscence is a surgical complication in which two sides of a surgical incision separate and rupture along the incision. Wound dehiscence risk factors include age, collagen-related disorders (e.g. Ehler-Danols syndrome), diabetes, obesity, poor suture knotting, and trauma to the surgical site. Wound dehiscence is estimated to occur in 0.5%–3.4% of abdominopelvic surgeries, and results in mortality in approximately 40% of cases [112]. Figs. 12.2 and 12.3 show wound dehiscence after surgery.

Wound Care Management and Early Treatment for Surgical Incisions

1. In case of infection, start antibiotic administration under medical supervision.
2. In case of wound dehiscence, leave the wound open and hospitalize the patient.
3. Clean the wound with isotonic saline other than water.
4. Cover the wound with sterile gauze and hospitalize the patient if needed.
5. Apply antiseptic solutions and provide appropriate wound dressing.

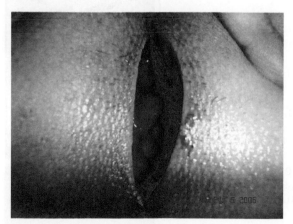

FIG. 12.1 A surgical incision with sharp edges after excision of a pilonidal sinus.

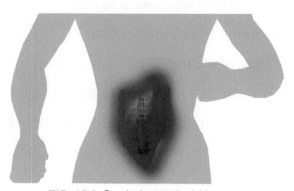

FIG. 12.2 Surgical wounds dehiscence.

Atlas of Wound Healing. https://doi.org/10.1016/B978-0-323-67968-8.00012-4

131

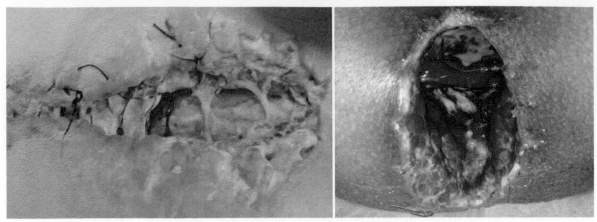

FIG. 12.3 Wound dehiscence due to infection.

Case Reports

Figs. 12.4—12.22 show the treatment process for traumatic wounds.

Surgical Incision

Year: 2018

Age and Sex: 58, F

Wound site: Abdominal region

Duration of treatment: 43 days

Cause of wound: Surgical incision dehiscence.

Treatment: Nano colloidal silver solution was used for wound disinfection. Sodium alginate and chitosan (gel and powder) were used for autolytic debridement and tissue regeneration, respectively.

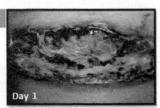

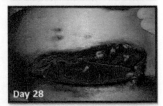

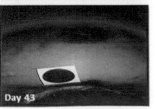

FIG. 12.4 Surgical incision.

Surgical Incision

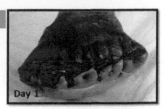

Year: 2018

Age and Sex: 73, F

Wound site: Right foot

Duration of treatment: 60 days

Cause of wound: Wound dehiscence after amputation.

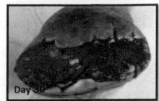

Treatment: Nano colloidal silver solution was used for wound disinfection. Sodium alginate was used for autolytic debridement. After removal of necrotic tissue, treatment was continued with chitosan gel and calcium alginate for tissue regeneration.

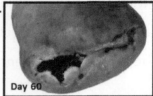

FIG. 12.5 Surgical incision.

Surgical Incision

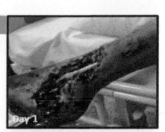

Year: 2018

Age and Sex: 29, M

Wound site: Left foot

Duration of treatment: 60 days

Cause of wound: Unsuccessful skin grafting after an accident.

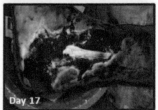

Treatment: Nano colloidal silver solution was used for wound disinfection. Chitosan gel and powder were used for tissue regeneration.

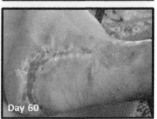

FIG. 12.6 Surgical incision.

Surgical Incision

Year: 2017

Age and Sex: 26, M

Wound site: Head

Duration of treatment: 15 days

Cause of wound: Unsuccessful primary suturing of a traumatic ulcer, developed to necrotic tissue.

Treatment: Nano colloidal silver solution was used for wound disinfection. Sodium alginate and chitosan gel were used for autolytic debridement and tissue regeneration, respectively.

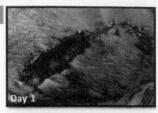
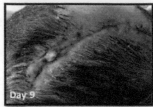
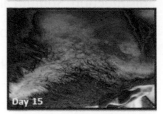

FIG. 12.7 Surgical incision.

Surgical Incision

Year: 2017

Age and Sex: 65, F

Wound site: Abdominal region

Duration of treatment: 29 days

Cause of wound: Infected incision site after oophorectomy.

Treatment: Nano colloidal silver solution was used for wound disinfection. Sodium alginate and chitosan gel were used for autolytic debridement and tissue regeneration, respectively.

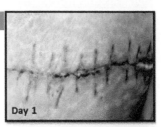
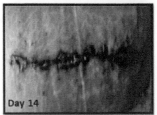
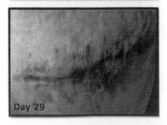

FIG. 12.8 Surgical incision.

Surgical Incision

Year: 2016

Age and Sex: 2.5, F

Wound site: Right foot

Duration of treatment: 60 days

Cause of wound: Removal of rhabdomyosarcoma tumor.

Treatment: Nano colloidal silver solution was used for wound disinfection. Chitosan gel and powder were applied for tissue regeneration.

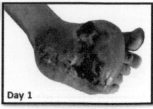
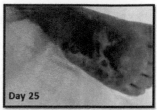
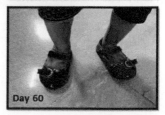

FIG. 12.9 Surgical incision.

Surgical Incision

Year: 2016

Age and Sex: 78, F

Wound site: Right leg

Duration of treatment: 25 days

Cause of wound: Infected incision site.

Treatment: Nano colloidal silver solution was used for wound disinfection. Sodium alginate and chitosan gel were used for autolytic debridement and tissue regeneration, respectively.

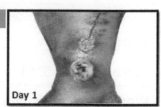
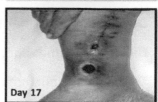
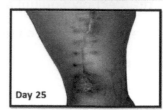

FIG. 12.10 Surgical incision.

Surgical Incision

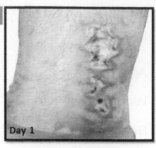
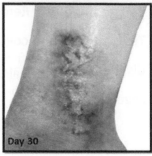

Year: 2015

Age and Sex: 14, F

Wound site: Left leg

Duration of treatment: 30 days

Cause of wound: Surgical incision dehiscence.

Treatment: Nano colloidal silver solution was used for wound disinfection. Sodium alginate and chitosan gel were used for autolytic debridement and tissue regeneration, respectively.

FIG. 12.11 Surgical incision.

Surgical Incision

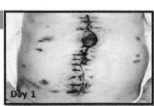
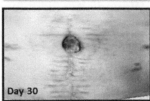
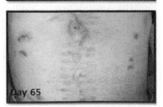

Year: 2015

Age and Sex: 45, M

Wound site: Abdominal region

Duration of treatment: 65 days

Cause of wound: Surgical incision dehiscence.

Treatment: Nano colloidal silver solution was used for wound disinfection. Sodium alginate and chitosan (gel and powder) were used for autolytic debridement and tissue regeneration, respectively.

FIG. 12.12 Surgical incision.

Surgical Incision

Year: 2015

Age and Sex: 34, M

Wound site: Gluteal region

Duration of treatment: 94 days

Cause of wound: Surgical wound dehiscence.

Treatment: Nano colloidal silver solution was used for wound disinfection. Chitosan gel and powder were used for tissue regeneration.

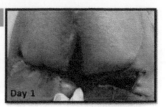
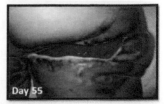
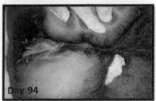
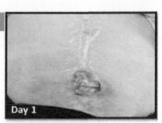

FIG. 12.13 Surgical incision.

Surgical Incision

Year: 2015

Age and Sex: 68, M

Wound site: Right trochanter

Duration of treatment: 35 days

Cause of wound: Surgical incision dehiscence.

Treatment: Nano colloidal silver solution was used for wound disinfection. Sodium alginate and chitosan (gel and powder) were used for autolytic debridement and tissue regeneration, respectively.

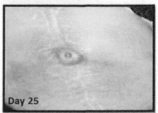
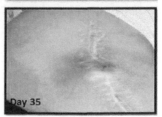

FIG. 12.14 Surgical incision.

Surgical Incision

Year: 2014

Age and Sex: 58, M

Wound site: Right big toe

Duration of treatment: 67 days

Cause of wound: Surgical incision dehiscence.

Treatment: Nano colloidal silver solution was used for wound disinfection. Sodium alginate and chitosan gel were used for autolytic debridement and tissue regeneration, respectively.

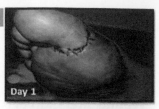
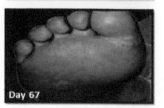
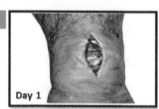

FIG. 12.15 Surgical incision.

Surgical Incision

Year: 2014

Age and Sex: 52, M

Wound site: Left leg

Duration of treatment: 24 days

Cause of wound: Surgical incision dehiscence.

Treatment: Nano colloidal silver solution was used for wound disinfection. Calcium alginate and chitosan gel were used for tissue regeneration.

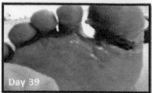
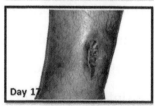
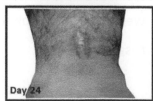

FIG. 12.16 Surgical incision.

Surgical Incision

Year: 2011

Age and Sex: 10, M

Wound site: Perineum

Duration of treatment: 27 days

Cause of wound: Surgical incision dehiscence.

Treatment: Nano colloidal silver solution was used for wound disinfection. Sodium alginate and chitosan powder were used for removal of slough tissue and tissue regeneration, respectively.

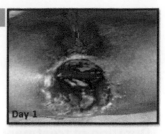
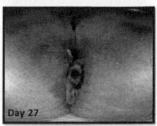

FIG. 12.17 Surgical incision.

Surgical Incision

Year: 2006

Age and Sex: 15, M

Wound site: Sacral region

Duration of treatment: 35 days

Cause of wound: Pilonidal cyctectomy.

Treatment: Nano colloidal silver solution was used for wound disinfection. Calcium alginate was applied for tissue regeneration.

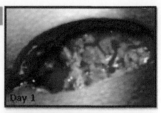
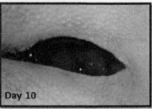
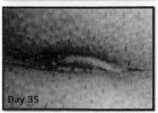

FIG. 12.18 Surgical incision.

Surgical Incision

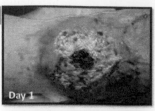

Year: 2006

Age and Sex: 75, F

Wound site: Left ankle

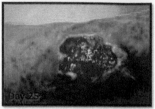

Duration of treatment: 55 days

Cause of wound: Unsuccessful grafting of an avulsion by car accident.

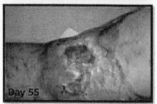

Treatment: Nano colloidal silver solution was used for wound disinfection. Sodium alginate was used for autolytic debridement of necrotic tissue and slough tissue, then treatment was continued with chitosan gel.

FIG. 12.19 Surgical incision.

Surgical Incision

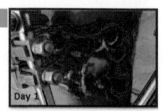

Year: 2006

Age and Sex: 18, M

Wound site: Right leg

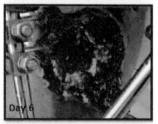

Duration of treatment: 14 days

Cause of wound: Infected wound dehiscence after surgical wound closure.

Treatment: Nano colloidal silver solution was used for wound disinfection. Sodium alginate was used for autolytic debridement of slough tissue, then treatment was continued with chitosan gel and powder.

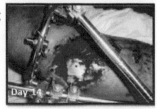

FIG. 12.20 Surgical incision.

Surgical Incision

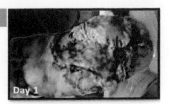

Year: 2006

Age and Sex: 19, M

Wound site: Right sole

Duration of treatment: 27 days (ready for skin graft)

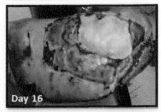

Cause of wound: Unsuccessful grafting of a traumatic wound caused by mine explosion.

Treatment: Nano colloidal silver solution was used for wound disinfection. Sodium alginate was used for autolytic debridement of necrotic tissue and slough tissue, then treatment was continued with chitosan gel and powder.

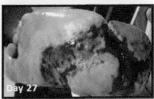

FIG. 12.21 Surgical incision.

Surgical Incision

Year: 2005

Age and Sex: 19, F

Wound site: Right leg

Duration of treatment: 53 days

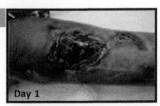

Cause of wound: Unsuccessful wound closure after knee surgery.

Treatment: Nano colloidal silver solution was used for wound disinfection. Sharp debridement along with sodium alginate were used for autolytic debridement, then treatment was continued with chitosan (gel and powder).

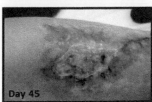

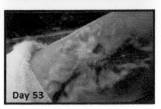

FIG. 12.22 Surgical incision.

CHAPTER 13

Atypical Wounds

Atypical wounds are commonly caused by uncommon etiologies with less prevalence compared to the other types of wounds. Inflammation disorders, infection, vasculopathies, metabolic disorders, genetic factors, malignancies, and external causes are the most common etiologies for atypical wounds.

Precise and multiple assessment techniques are required before diagnosis and management of atypical wounds including family history, personal habits, systemic disease, and physical examination [22].

There are many types of atypical wounds such as malignant ulcers, pemphigus vulgaris, pyoderma gangrenosum, necrobiosis lipoidica, epidermolysis bullosa, antiphospholipid Syndrome, Raynaud's phenomenon, Buerger's Disease, calciphylaxis and Iatrogenic factors, and drug. The major types are mentioned as follows:

MALIGNANT ULCERS

Most malignant ulcers are the results of a primary malignancy; however, a tumor can metastase to the epidermal tissue. In total, 6%—19% of patients with cancer experience malignant ulcers. These ulcers grow rapidly, emerge to the surrounding tissues, and result in fistula or sinus (Fig. 13.1).

PYODERMA GANGRENOSUM

Patients usually give a history of painful pustules with erythema, after trauma, which rupture and ulcerate at trauma site.

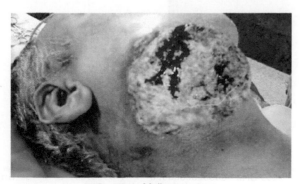

FIG. 13.1 Malignant ulcer.

Atlas of Wound Healing. https://doi.org/10.1016/B978-0-323-67968-8.00013-6

The diagnosis of pyoderma gangrenosum is primarily clinical, but histological experiments may be needed. The ulcer is characterized by painful erythema or violaceous raised edge in venipuncture. The wound bed is often purulent and may extend to muscle. Surgical debridement is contraindicated to prevent the ulcer from worsening and complications. Immunosuppressive are recommended for treatment [39,113].

NECROBIOSIS LIPOIDICA

Necrobiosis lipoidica (NL) is a rare, chronic, idiopathic, granulomatous disease of collagen degeneration, which leads to a pretibial yellowish atrophic plaque. It often occurs in patients with diabetes mellitus (usually type 1), but it can also be associated with rheumatoid arthritis.

These types of ulcers are sores that heal slowly, and the possibility of infection is high.

They can be healed by using topical corticosteroids [114].

PEMPHIGUS VULGARIS

Pemphigus is an autoimmune blistering disease that affects skin and mucous membrane and usually occurs in adults with a mean age of 40—60 years. The incidence of pemphigus ranges from 0.1 to 0.5/100,000 per year. In Iran, the incidence rate is estimated approximately 5/100,000. The common manifestations of the disease are painful erosions in oral mucosa and flaccid blisters on the normal skin or erythematous base [115,116] (Fig. 13.2).

EB WOUNDS

Epidermolysis bullosa (EB) is an inherited rare genetic connective tissue disorder caused by keratinocytes malfunction, which results in extremely fragile skin and blistering after minimal trauma. EB is characterized by painful skin/mucosal lesions, nail dystrophy, and alopecia. Skin lesions heal without scarring while blistering decreases with age [117—119] (Fig. 13.3).

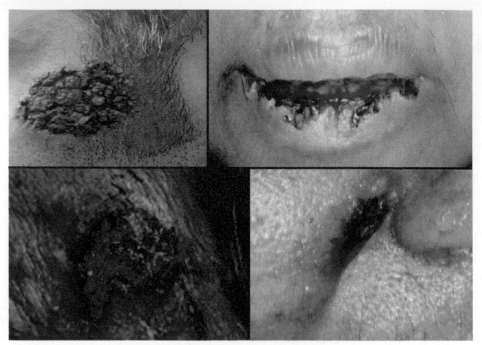

FIG. 13.2 Pemphigus vulgaris ulcer.

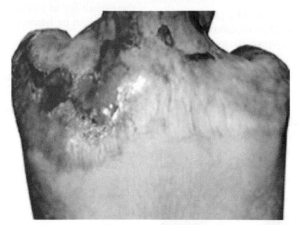

FIG. 13.3 EB wound.

Case Reports

Figs. 13.4–13.28 show the treatment process for atypical wounds.

Atypical Wound

Year: 2018

Age and Sex: 41, F

Wound site: Shoulder

Duration of treatment: 40 days

Cause of wound: Drained abscess caused by infected injection site.

Treatment: Nano colloidal silver solution was used for wound disinfection. Sodium alginate and chitosan (gel and powder) were used for autolytic removal of slough tissue and tissue regeneration, respectively.

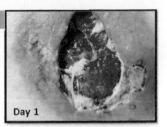
Day 1

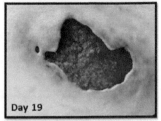
Day 19

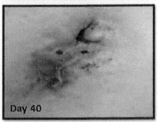
Day 40

FIG. 13.4 Atypical wound.

Atypical Wound

Year: 2018

Age and Sex: 28, F

Wound site: Hands

Duration of treatment: 10 days

Cause of wound: Unknown allergy.

Treatment: Nano colloidal silver solution was used for wound disinfection. Chitosan gel was applied for the treatment.

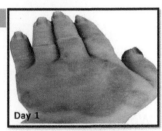
Day 1

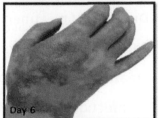
Day 6

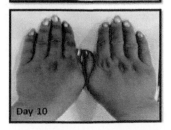
Day 10

FIG. 13.5 Atypical wound.

Atypical Wound

Year: 2018

Age and Sex: 54, F

Wound site: Right hand

Duration of treatment: 5 days

Cause of wound: Idiopathic blisters.

Treatment: Nano colloidal silver solution was used for wound disinfection. After sharp removal of blisters, chitosan gel was applied for tissue regeneration.

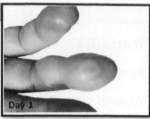
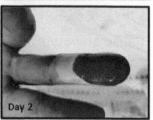
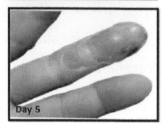

FIG. 13.6 Atypical wound.

Atypical Wound

Year: 2017

Age and Sex: 67, F

Wound site: Right hand

Duration of treatment: 93 days

Cause of wound: Chemotherapy infusion.

Treatment: Nano colloidal silver solution was used for wound disinfection. Sodium alginate was used for autolytic debridement of yellow slough tissue, then treatment was continued with chitosan gel and powder.

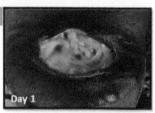
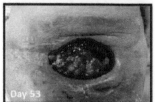
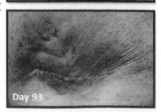

FIG. 13.7 Atypical wound.

Atypical Wound

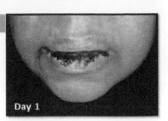

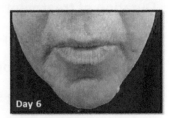

Year: 2017

Age and Sex: 52, F

Wound site: Lips

Duration of treatment: 6 days

Cause of wound: Pemphigus vulgaris blisters.

Treatment: Silver nanoparticle gel was used to disinfect the wound then activating tissue regeneration.

FIG. 13.8 Atypical wound.

Atypical Wound

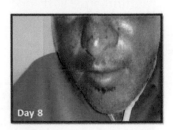

Year: 2017

Age and Sex: 25, M

Wound site: Nose

Duration of treatment: 8 days

Cause of wound: Pemphigus vulgaris blisters.

Treatment: Silver nanoparticle gel was used to disinfect the wound then activating tissue regeneration.

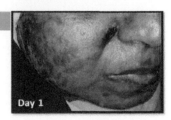

FIG. 13.9 Atypical wound.

Atypical Wound

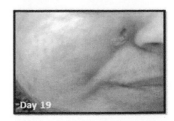

Year: 2017

Age and Sex: 52, F

Wound site: Face

Duration of treatment: 19 days

Cause of wound: Pemphigus vulgaris blisters.

Treatment: Silver nanoparticle gel was used to disinfect the wound then activating tissue regeneration.

FIG. 13.10 Atypical wound.

Atypical Wound

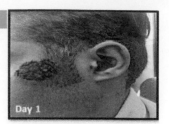

Year: 2017

Age and Sex: 27, M

Wound site: Face

Duration of treatment: 45 days

Cause of wound: Pemphigus vulgaris blisters.

Treatment: Silver nanoparticle gel was used to disinfect the wound then activating tissue regeneration.

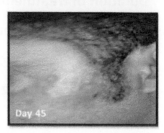

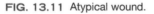
FIG. 13.11 Atypical wound.

Atypical Wound

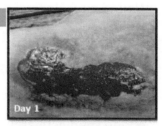

Year: 2017

Age and Sex: 60, M

Wound site: Shoulder

Duration of treatment: 37 days

Cause of wound: Pemphigus vulgaris blisters.

Treatment: Silver nanoparticle gel was used to disinfect the wound then activating tissue regeneration.

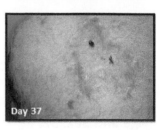

FIG. 13.12 Atypical wound.

Atypical Wound

Year: 2017

Age and Sex: 45, M

Wound site: Face

Duration of treatment: 28 days

Cause of wound: Pemphigus vulgaris blisters.

Treatment: Silver nanoparticle gel was used to disinfect the wound then activating tissue regeneration.

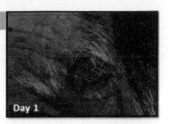
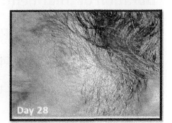

FIG. 13.13 Atypical wound.

Atypical Wound

Year: 2017

Age and Sex: 62, M

Wound site: Head

Duration of treatment: 33 days

Cause of wound: Pemphigus vulgaris blisters.

Treatment: Silver nanoparticle gel was used to disinfect the wound then activating tissue regeneration.

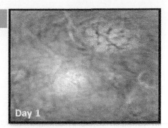
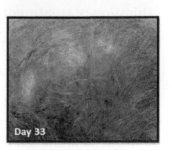

FIG. 13.14 Atypical wound.

Atypical Wound

Year: 2017

Age and Sex: 32, M

Wound site: Nose

Duration of treatment: 30 days

Cause of wound: Pemphigus vulgaris blisters.

Treatment: Silver nanoparticle gel was used to disinfect the wound then activating tissue regeneration.

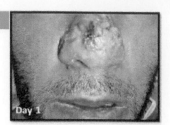
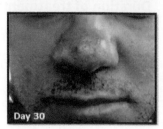

FIG. 13.15 Atypical wound.

Atypical Wound

Year: 2017

Age and Sex: 63, M

Wound site: Back region

Duration of treatment: 18 days

Cause of wound: Pemphigus vulgaris blisters.

Treatment: Silver nanoparticle gel was used to disinfect the wound then activating tissue regeneration.

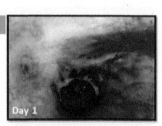
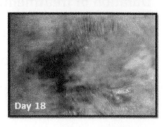

FIG. 13.16 Atypical wound.

Atypical Wound

Year: 2017

Age and Sex: 32, M

Wound site: Face

Duration of treatment: 21 days

Cause of wound: Pemphigus vulgaris blisters.

Treatment: Silver nanoparticle gel was used to disinfect the wound then activating tissue regeneration.

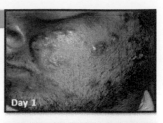
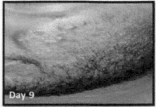
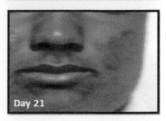
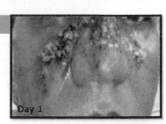

FIG. 13.17 Atypical wound.

Atypical Wound

Year: 2017

Age and Sex: 46, M

Wound site: Face

Duration of treatment: 8 days

Cause of wound: Pemphigus vulgaris blisters.

Treatment: Silver nanoparticle gel was used to disinfect the wound then activating tissue regeneration.

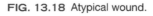
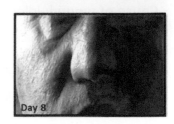

FIG. 13.18 Atypical wound.

Atypical Wound

Year: 2017

Age and Sex: 46, M

Wound site: Face

Duration of treatment: 47 days

Cause of wound: Pemphigus vulgaris blisters.

Treatment: Silver nanoparticle gel was used to disinfect the wound then activating tissue regeneration.

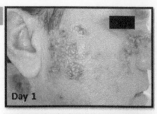
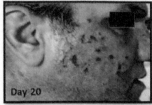
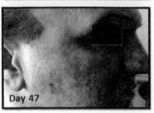

FIG. 13.19 Atypical wound.

Atypical Wound

Year: 2017

Age and Sex: 73, F

Wound site: Left thigh

Duration of treatment: 37days

Cause of wound: Idiopathic blister which developed to a chronic ulcer.

Treatment: Nano colloidal silver solution was used for wound disinfection. Sodium alginate was applied to remove fibrotic tissue and chitosan gel was applied for tissue regeneration.

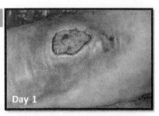
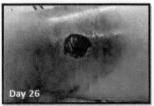
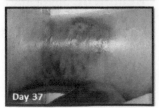

FIG. 13.20 Atypical wound.

Atypical Wound

Year: 2016

Age and Sex: 45, M

Wound site: Right thigh

Duration of treatment: 75 days

Cause of wound: Idiopathic ulcer

Treatment: Nano colloidal silver solution was used for wound disinfection. After sharp debridement of wound edges, sodium alginate and chitosan gel were used for autolytic debridement and tissue regeneration, respectively.

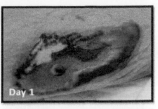
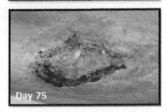
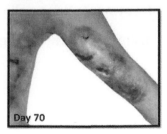

FIG. 13.21 Atypical wound.

Atypical Wound

Year: 2015

Age and Sex: 14, F

Wound site: Right hand

Duration of treatment: 70 days

Cause of wound: Epidermolysis bullosa (EB)

Treatment: Nano colloidal silver solution was used for wound disinfection. Chitosan gel was applied for tissue regeneration.

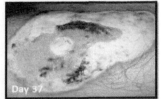
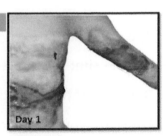

FIG. 13.22 Atypical wound.

Atypical Wound

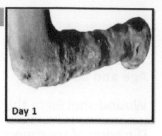

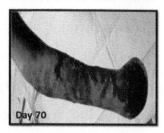

Year: 2015

Age and Sex: 14, F

Wound site: Right hand

Duration of treatment: 70 days

Cause of wound: Epidermolysis bullosa (EB)

Treatment: Nano colloidal silver solution was used for wound disinfection. Chitosan gel was applied for tissue regeneration.

FIG. 13.23 Atypical wound.

Atypical Wound

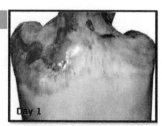

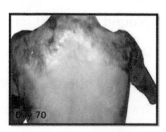

Year: 2015

Age and Sex: 14, F

Wound site: Shoulders

Duration of treatment: 70 days

Cause of wound: Epidermolysis bullosa (EB)

Treatment: Nano colloidal silver solution was used for wound disinfection. Chitosan gel was applied for tissue regeneration.

FIG. 13.24 Atypical wound.

Atypical Wound

Year: 2007

Age and Sex: 55, F

Wound site: Left side of neck

Duration of treatment: 5 days

Cause of wound: Burn caused by radiotherapy

Treatment: Nano colloidal silver solution was used for wound disinfection. Chitosan gel was applied for tissue regeneration.

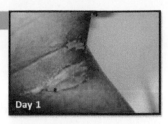
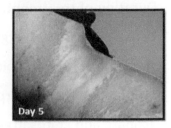

FIG. 13.25 Atypical wound.

Atypical Wound

Year: 2005

Age and Sex: 14, M

Wound site: Left heel

Duration of treatment: 16 days

Cause of wound: Dominant multiple sensory neuropathy

Treatment: Nano colloidal silver solution was used for wound disinfection. Sodium alginate and chitosan gel were used for autolytic debridement and tissue regeneration, respectively.

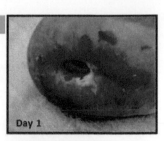
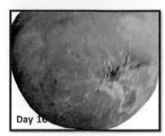

FIG. 13.26 Atypical wound.

Atypical Wound

Year: 2005

Age and Sex: 11, F

Wound site: Lateral side of right leg

Duration of treatment: 45 days

Cause of wound: Allergy to orthopedic cast

Treatment: Nano colloidal silver solution was used for wound disinfection. After sharp debridement of wound edges, sodium alginate and chitosan gel were used for autolytic debridement and tissue regeneration, respectively.

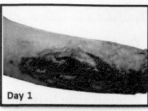
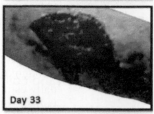
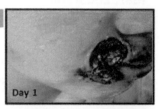

FIG. 13.27 Atypical wound.

Atypical Wound

Year: 2005

Age and Sex: 13, F

Wound site: Lips

Duration of treatment: 17 days

Cause of wound: Necrotic ulcer caused by Herpes in a cancerous patient.

Treatment: Nano colloidal silver solution was used for wound disinfection. After sharp debridement of wound edges, sodium alginate and chitosan gel were used for autolytic debridement and tissue regeneration, respectively.

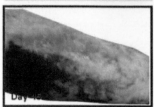
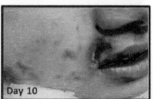
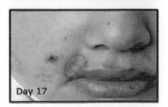

FIG. 13.28 Atypical wound.

References

[1] A. Rahmani Del Bakhshayesh, N. Annabi, R. Khalilov, A. Akbarzadeh, M. Samiei, E. Alizadeh, M. Alizadeh-Ghodsi, S. Davaran, A. Montaseri, Recent advances on biomedical applications of scaffolds in wound healing and dermal tissue engineering, Artif. Cells. Nanomed. Biotechnol. 46 (2018) 691–705.

[2] N. Bhardwaj, D. Chouhan, B. B Mandal, Tissue engineered skin and wound healing: current strategies and future directions, Curr. Pharmaceut. Des. 23 (2017) 3455–3482.

[3] S.-K. Han, Innovations and Advances in Wound Healing, Springer, 2015.

[4] F.-M. Chen, X. Liu, Advancing biomaterials of human origin for tissue engineering, Prog. Polym. Sci. 53 (2016) 86–168.

[5] S.R. Nussbaum, M.J. Carter, C.E. Fife, J. DaVanzo, R. Haught, M. Nusgart, D. Cartwright, An economic evaluation of the impact, cost, and medicare policy implications of chronic nonhealing wounds, Value Health 21 (2018) 27–32.

[6] Cambridge Dictionary, Cambridge University Press; 2016, http://dictionary.cambridge.org/ru/ (дата обращения: 12.02.2016), (2017).

[7] R.I. Freshney, Culture of Animal Cells: A Manual of Basic Technique and Specialized Applications, John Wiley & Sons, 2015.

[8] W. Lopez-Ojeda, W.D. James, Anatomy, Skin (Integument), 2017.

[9] L. Klosterman, Skin.

[10] M. Ågren, Wound Healing Biomaterials-Volume 1: Therapies and Regeneration, Woodhead Publishing, 2016.

[11] M. Venus, J. Waterman, I. McNab, Basic physiology of the skin, Surgery (Oxford Int. Ed.) 28 (2010) 469–472.

[12] G.W. Jenkins, C.P. Kemnitz, G.J. Tortora, Anatomy and Physiology: From Science to Life, Wiley Hoboken, 2007.

[13] H. Shimizu, Shimizu's Textbook of Dermatology, Hokkaido University, 2007.

[14] J.G. Tidball, Mechanisms of muscle injury, repair, and regeneration, Compr. Physiol. 1 (2011) 2029–2062.

[15] K. Rogers, Skin and Connective Tissue, Britannica Educational Publishing, 2011.

[16] R. Florencio-Silva, G.R.d.S. Sasso, E. Sasso-Cerri, M.J. Simões, P.S. Cerri, Biology of bone tissue: structure, function, and factors that influence bone cells, BioMed. Res. Int. (2015).

[17] A. DeFranzo, L. Argenta, M. Marks, J. Molnar, L. David, L. Webb, W. Ward, R. Teasdall, The use of vacuum-assisted closure therapy for the treatment of lower-extremity wounds with exposed bone, Plast. Reconstr. Surg. 108 (2001) 1184–1191.

[18] P.A. Kolarsick, M.A. Kolarsick, C. Goodwin, Anatomy and physiology of the skin, J. Dermatol. Nurses. Assoc. 3 (2011) 203–213.

[19] G. Said, Peripheral Neuropathy & Neuropathic Pain: Into the Light, TFM Publishing Limited, 2014.

[20] J. Vuolo, Wound Care Made Incredibly Easy, Lippincott, Williams and Wilkins, 2009.

[21] W.M. Reichert, Indwelling Neural Implants: Strategies for Contending with the In Vivo Environment, CRC Press, 2007.

[22] S. Baranoski, E.A. Ayello, Wound Care Essentials: Practice Principles, Lippincott Williams & Wilkins, 2008.

[23] S. Barrientos, O. Stojadinovic, M.S. Golinko, H. Brem, M. Tomic-Canic, Growth factors and cytokines in wound healing, Wound Repair Regen. 16 (2008) 585–601.

[24] S.F. Swaim, D.M. Bradley, S.H. Hinkle, Wound contraction: basic and clinical factors, Compendium on Continuing Education For The Practising Veterinarian-North American Edition 23 (2001) 20–35.

[25] M.P. Caley, V.L. Martins, E.A. O'Toole, Metalloproteinases and wound healing, Adv. Wound Care 4 (2015) 225–234.

[26] M. Xue, C.J. Jackson, Extracellular matrix reorganization during wound healing and its impact on abnormal scarring, Adv. Wound Care 4 (2015) 119–136.

[27] World Report on Ageing and Health, World Health Organization, 2015.

[28] R. Sgonc, J. Gruber, Age-related aspects of cutaneous wound healing: a mini-review, Gerontology 59 (2013) 159–164.

[29] K. Anderson, R.L. Hamm, Factors that impair wound healing, J. Am. Coll. Clin. Wound Spec. 4 (2012) 84–91.

[30] S.a. Guo, L.A. DiPietro, Factors affecting wound healing, J. Dent. Res. 89 (2010) 219–229.

[31] K.L. Brown, T.J. Phillips, Nutrition and wound healing, Clin. Dermatol. 28 (2010) 432–439.

[32] D. Smith, R. Lane, R. McGinnes, J. O'Brien, R. Johnston, L. Bugeja, V. Team, C. Weller, What is the effect of exercise on wound healing in patients with venous leg ulcers? A systematic review, Int. Wound J. (2018) 441–453.

[33] J. O'brien, K. Finlayson, G. Kerr, H. Edwards, Evaluating the effectiveness of a self-management exercise intervention on wound healing, functional ability and health-related quality of life outcomes in adults with venous leg ulcers: a randomised controlled trial, Int. Wound J. 14 (2017) 130–137.

[34] T. Keylock, L. Meserve, A. Wolfe, Low-intensity exercise accelerates wound healing in diabetic mice, Wounds 30 (2018) 68–71.

[35] J. Goh, W.C. Ladiges, Exercise enhances wound healing and prevents cancer progression during aging by targeting macrophage polarity, Mech. Ageing Dev. 139 (2014) 41–48.

[36] B.D. Pence, J.A. Woods, Exercise, obesity, and cutaneous wound healing: evidence from rodent and human studies, Adv. Wound Care 3 (2014) 71–79.

[37] K. Izadi, P. Ganchi, Chronic wounds, Clin. Plast. Surg. 32 (2005) 209–222.

[38] C.T. Hess, Checklist for factors affecting wound healing, Adv. Skin Wound Care 24 (2011) 192.

[39] M.E. Edmonds, A. Foster, ABC of wound healing: diabetic foot ulcers, BMJ 332 (2006) 407.

[40] A. Jibawi, M. Baguneid, A. Bhowmick, Current Surgical Guidelines, Oxford University Press, 2018.

[41] J. Murtagh, John Murtagh's General Practice [Electronic Resource], McGraw-Hill, North Ryde, NSW, 2011.

[42] Y.J. Jun, D. Shin, W.J. Choi, J.H. Hwang, H. Kim, T.G. Kim, H.B. Lee, T.S. Oh, H.W. Shin, H.S. Suh, A mobile application for wound assessment and treatment: findings of a user trial, Int. J. Low. Extrem. Wounds 15 (2016) 344–353.

[43] S.C. Wang, J.A. Anderson, R. Evans, K. Woo, B. Beland, D. Sasseville, L. Moreau, Point-of-care wound visioning technology: reproducibility and accuracy of a wound measurement app, PLoS One 12 (2017) e0183139.

[44] B.A. Lipsky, C. Hoey, Topical antimicrobial therapy for treating chronic wounds, Clin. Infect. Dis. 49 (2009) 1541–1549.

[45] S. Kordestani, F. NayebHabib, M.H. Saadatjo, A novel wound rinsing solution based on nano colloidal silver, Nanomed. J. 1 (2014) 315–323.

[46] Y. Oka, T. Kuroshima, K. Sawachika, M. Yamashita, M. Sakao, K. Ohnishi, K. Asami, M. Yatsuzuka, Preparation of silver nanocolloidal solution by cavitation bubble plasma, Vacuum (2018). Article in press.

[47] G. Franci, A. Falanga, S. Galdiero, L. Palomba, M. Rai, G. Morelli, M. Galdiero, Silver nanoparticles as potential antibacterial agents, Molecules 20 (2015) 8856–8874.

[48] A. Nauta, G. Gurtner, M. Longaker, Wound healing and regenerative strategies, Oral Dis. 17 (2011) 541–549.

[49] A. Bhatia, Epidermal skin grafting in patients with complex wounds: a case series, J. Wound Care 25 (2016) 148–153.

[50] A. Andreassi, R. Bilenchi, M. Biagioli, C. D'Aniello, Classification and pathophysiology of skin grafts, Clin. Dermatol. 23 (2005) 332–337.

[51] J.K. Robinson, C.W. Hanke, D.M. Siegel, A. Fratila, A.C. Bhatia, T.E. Rohrer, Surgery of the Skin E-Book: Procedural Dermatology, Elsevier Health Sciences, 2014.

[52] R. Shimizu, K. Kishi, Skin graft, Plastic Surg. Int. (2012).

[53] H. Schubert, M. Brandstetter, F. Ensat, H. Kohlosy, A. Schwabegger, Split thickness skin graft for coverage of soft tissue defects, Operat. Orthop. Traumatol. 24 (2012) 432–438.

[54] S. Kanji, H. Das, Advances of Stem Cell Therapeutics in Cutaneous Wound Healing and Regeneration, Mediators of inflammation, 2017.

[55] V. Falanga, Stem cells in tissue repair and regeneration, J. Invest. Dermatol. 132 (2012) 1538–1541.

[56] C.A. Herberts, M.S. Kwa, H.P. Hermsen, Risk factors in the development of stem cell therapy, J. Transl. Med. 9 (2011) 29.

[57] V. Singh, R. Singh, Platelet rich plasma—a new revolution in medicine, J. Anat. Soc. India (2017) S28–S30.

[58] K.M. Lacci, A. Dardik, Platelet-rich plasma: support for its use in wound healing, Yale J. Biol. Med. 83 (2010) 1.

[59] P. Rousselle, F. Braye, G. Dayan, Re-epithelialization of Adult Skin Wounds: Cellular Mechanisms and Therapeutic Strategies, Advanced drug delivery reviews, 2018.

[60] K. Kothari, Role of platelet-rich plasma: the current trend and evidence, Indian J. Pain 31 (2017) 1.

[61] E. Fitzpatrick, O.J. Holland, J.J. Vanderlelie, Ozone therapy for the treatment of chronic wounds: a systematic review, Int. Wound J. (2018) 633–644.

[62] A.M. Fathi, M.N. Mawsouf, R. Viebahn-Hänsler, Ozone therapy in diabetic foot and chronic, nonhealing wounds, Ozone: Sci. Eng. 34 (2012) 438–450.

[63] M. Mutluoglu, A. Cakkalkurt, G. Uzun, S. Aktas, Topical oxygen for chronic wounds: a PRO/CON debate, J. Am. Coll. Clin. Wound Spec. 5 (2013) 61–65.

[64] V. Agarwal, S. Aroor, N. Gupta, A. Gupta, N. Agarwal, N. Kaur, New technique of applying topical oxygen therapy as a cost-effective procedure, Indian J. Surg. 77 (2015) 1456–1459.

[65] J.W. van Neck, B. Tuk, E.M. Fijneman, J.J. Redeker, E.M. Talahatu, M. Tong, Hyperbaric oxygen therapy for wound healing in diabetic rats: varying efficacy after a clinically-based protocol, PLoS One 12 (2017) e0177766.

[66] P. Kranke, M.H. Bennett, M.-S. James, A. Schnabel, S.E. Debus, S. Weibel, Hyperbaric oxygen therapy for chronic wounds, Cochrane Database Syst. Rev. 6 (2015).

[67] P.M. Tibbles, J.S. Edelsberg, Hyperbaric-oxygen therapy, N. Engl. J. Med. 334 (1996) 1642–1648.

[68] P.S. Nain, S.K. Uppal, R. Garg, K. Bajaj, S. Garg, Role of negative pressure wound therapy in healing of diabetic foot ulcers, J. Surg. Tech. Case Rep. 3 (2011).

[69] B.J. Stanley, Negative pressure wound therapy, Vet Clin. Small Anim. Prac. 47 (2017) 1203–1220.

[70] R. Samaneh, Y. Ali, J. Mostafa, N.A. Mahmud, R. Zohre, Laser therapy for wound healing: a review of current techniques and mechanisms of action, Biosci. Biotech. Res. Asia 12 (2015) 217–223.

[71] B.M. Kajagar, A.S. Godhi, A. Pandit, S. Khatri, Efficacy of low level laser therapy on wound healing in patients with chronic diabetic foot ulcers—a randomised control trial, Indian J. Surg. 74 (2012) 359–363.

[72] J. Zuccaro, N. Ziolkowski, J. Fish, A systematic review of the effectiveness of laser therapy for hypertrophic burn scars, Clin. Plast. Surg. 44 (2017) 767–779.

[73] C. Starkey, Therapeutic Modalities, Chapter 11: Low Laser Therapy, fourth ed., F.A. Davis, 2013.

[74] A.M. Smith, S. Moxon, G. Morris, Biopolymers as Wound Healing Materials, Wound Healing Biomaterials, Elsevier, 2016, pp. 261–287.

[75] D.B. Doughty, L.L. McNichol, Wound, Ostomy, and Continence Nurses Society Core Curriculum: Wound Management, Wolters Kluwer, 2015.

[76] S.S. Kordestani, Natural Biopolymers: Wound Care Applications, Encyclopedia of Biomedical Polymers and Polymeric Biomaterials, 2014, pp. 1–14.

[77] B.A. Myers, Wound Management: Principles and Practice, Pearson/Prentice Hall, 2008.

[78] C.D. Marshall, M.S. Hu, T. Leavitt, L.A. Barnes, H.P. Lorenz, M.T. Longaker, Cutaneous scarring: basic science, current treatments, and future directions, Adv. Wound Care 7 (2018) 29–45.

[79] A.D. Rodrigues, Scarless Wound Healing, CRC Press, 2016.

[80] S. Monstrey, E. Middelkoop, J.J. Vranckx, F. Bassetto, U.E. Ziegler, S. Meaume, L. Téot, Updated scar management practical guidelines: non-invasive and invasive measures, J. Plast. Reconstr. Aesthetic Surg. 67 (2014) 1017–1025.

[81] G.G. Gauglitz, H.C. Korting, T. Pavicic, T. Ruzicka, M.G. Jeschke, Hypertrophic scarring and keloids: pathomechanisms and current and emerging treatment strategies, Mol. Med. 17 (2011) 113.

[82] A. Bayat, D. McGrouther, M. Ferguson, Skin scarring, BMJ 326 (2003) 88.

[83] N.J. Percival, Classification of wounds and their management, Surgery (Oxford) 20 (2002) 114–117.

[84] S. Dhivya, V.V. Padma, E. Santhini, Wound dressings—a review, Biomedicine 5 (2015).

[85] C.K. Lee, S.L. Hansen, Management of acute wounds, Surg. Clin. 89 (2009) 659–676.

[86] J. Weinzweig, Plastic Surgery Secrets Plus E-Book, Elsevier Health Sciences, 2010.

[87] S. Barrientos, H. Brem, O. Stojadinovic, M. Tomic-Canic, Clinical application of growth factors and cytokines in wound healing, Wound Repair Regen. 22 (2014) 569–578.

[88] M. Gray, National Pressure Ulcer Advisory Panel (NPUAP), NPUAP pressure injury stages, in: NPUAP 2016 Staging Consensus Conference, Chicago, 2016. http://www.npuap.org/resources/educational-and-clinical-resources/npuap-pressure-injury-stages/.

[89] S. Noor, M. Zubair, J. Ahmad, Diabetic foot ulcer—a review on pathophysiology, classification and microbial etiology, Diabetes Metab. Syndr. Clin. Res. Rev. 9 (2015) 192–199.

[90] IDF Diabetes Atlas, 2017.

[91] Z. Punthakee, R. Goldenberg, P. Katz, D.C.C.P.G.E. Committee, Definition, classification and diagnosis of diabetes, prediabetes and metabolic syndrome, Can. J. Diabetes 42 (2018) S10–S15.

[92] K.T. Kwon, D.G. Armstrong, Microbiology and antimicrobial therapy for diabetic foot infections, Infect. Chemother. 50 (2018) 11–20.

[93] E. Everett, N. Mathioudakis, Update on management of diabetic foot ulcers, Ann. N. Y. Acad. Sci. 1411 (2018) 153–165.

[94] A. Alavi, R.G. Sibbald, D. Mayer, L. Goodman, M. Botros, D.G. Armstrong, K. Woo, T. Boeni, E.A. Ayello, R.S. Kirsner, Diabetic foot ulcers: Part I. Pathophysiology and prevention, J. Am. Acad. Dermatol. 70 (2014) 1.e1–1.e18.

[95] Z. Iqbal, S. Azmi, R. Yadav, M. Ferdousi, M. Kumar, D.J. Cuthbertson, J. Lim, R.A. Malik, U. Alam, Diabetic Peripheral Neuropathy: Epidemiology, Diagnosis, and Pharmacotherapy, Clinical Therapeutics, 2018.

[96] L.j. Yan, Redox imbalance stress in diabetes mellitus: role of the polyol pathway, Animal Models Exp. Med. 1 (2018) 7–13.

[97] D.G. Armstrong, A.J. Boulton, S.A. Bus, Diabetic foot ulcers and their recurrence, N. Engl. J. Med. 376 (2017) 2367–2375.

[98] S. Singh, D.R. Pai, C. Yuhhui, Diabetic foot ulcer—diagnosis and management, Clin. Res. Foot. Ankle. 1 (2013) 120.

[99] P. Altmeyer, K. Hoffmann, S. el Gammal, J. Hutchinson, Wound Healing and Skin Physiology, Springer Science & Business Media, 2012.

[100] M. Dąbrowski, J. Lewandowski, P. Abramczyk, I. Łoń, Z. Gaciong, M. Siński, Atrial fibrillation does not affect ankle–brachial index measured using the Doppler method, Hypertens. Res. 41 (2018) 60.

[101] A. Oryan, E. Alemzadeh, A. Moshiri, Burn wound healing: present concepts, treatment strategies and future directions, J. Wound Care 26 (2017) 5–19.

[102] V. Tiwari, Burn wound: how it differs from other wounds? Indian J. Plast. Surg. 45 (2012) 364.

[103] T. Schaefer, K. Szymanski, Burns, Evaluation And Management, 2017.

[104] R.A. Moore, B. Burns, Rule of Nines, StatPearls [Internet], StatPearls Publishing, 2018.

[105] J.E. Grey, K.G. Harding, S. Enoch, Venous and arterial leg ulcers, BMJ 332 (2006) 347–350.

[106] J-h. Yue, S-j. Zhang, Q. Sun, Z-r. Sun, X-x. Wang, B. Golianu, Y. Lu, Q. Zhang, Local warming therapy for treating chronic wounds: a systematic review, Medicine 97 (2018).

[107] W.L. Olszewski, Lymphatic Ulcer of Lower Limb, Ulcers of the Lower Extremity, Springer, 2016, pp. 259–265.

[108] V.M. Karnasula, Management of ulcers in lymphoedematous limbs, Indian J. Plast. Surg. 45 (2012) 261.

[109] D.J. Leaper, ABC of wound healing: traumatic and surgical wounds, BMJ 332 (2006) 532.

[110] M. Jaindl, G. Oberleitner, G. Endler, C. Thallinger, F.M. Kovar, Management of bite wounds in children and adults—an analysis of over 5000 cases at a level I trauma centre, Wien. Klin. Wochenschr. 128 (2016) 367–375.

[111] D.W. Bratzler, E.P. Dellinger, K.M. Olsen, T.M. Perl, P.G. Auwaerter, M.K. Bolon, D.N. Fish, L.M. Napolitano, R.G. Sawyer, D. Slain, Clinical practice guidelines for antimicrobial prophylaxis in surgery, Surg. Infect. 14 (2013) 73—156.

[112] V.K. Shanmugam, S.J. Fernandez, K.K. Evans, S. McNish, A.N. Banerjee, K.S. Couch, M. Mete, N. Shara, Postoperative wound dehiscence: predictors and associations, Wound Repair Regen. 23 (2015) 184—190.

[113] N.S. Barbosa, S.N. Tolkachjov, R.A. el-Azhary, M.D. Davis, M.J. Camilleri, M.T. McEvoy, A.G. Bridges, D.A. Wetter, Clinical features, causes, treatments, and outcomes of peristomal pyoderma gangrenosum (PPG) in 44 patients: the Mayo Clinic experience, 1996 through 2013, J. Am. Acad. Dermatol. 75 (2016) 931—939.

[114] V. Mitre, C. Wang, R. Hunt, Necrobiosis Lipoidica, J. Pediatr. 179 (2016) 272—272.e271.

[115] F. Mokhtari, M. Matin, F. Rajati, Pemphigus vulgaris and amyotrophic lateral sclerosis, J. Res. Med. Sci. (2016) 21.

[116] M. Kasperkiewicz, C.T. Ellebrecht, H. Takahashi, J. Yamagami, D. Zillikens, A.S. Payne, M. Amagai, Pemphigus, Nat. Rev. Dis. Primers 3 (2017) 17026.

[117] E. Rashidghamat, J.A. McGrath, Novel and emerging therapies in the treatment of recessive dystrophic epidermolysis bullosa, Intractable Rare Dis. Res. 6 (2017) 6—20.

[118] V.L.S.Y. Boeira, E.S. Souza, B.d.O. Rocha, P.D. Oliveira, M.d.F.S.P. Oliveira, V.R.P.d.A. Rêgo, I. Follador, Inherited epidermolysis bullosa: clinical and therapeutic aspects, An. Bras. Dermatol. 88 (2013) 185—198.

[119] E. Pope, I. Lara-Corrales, J.E. Mellerio, A.E. Martinez, C. Sibbald, R.G. Sibbald, Epidermolysis bullosa and chronic wounds: a model for wound bed preparation of fragile skin, Adv. Skin Wound Care 26 (2013) 177—188.

Index

Note: Page numbers followed by "f" indicate figures, "t" indicate tables.

Printed and bound by CPI Group (UK) Ltd, Croydon, CR0 4YY

09/10/2024

01042653-0001